Books should be returned to the SDH Library on or before
the date stamped above unless a renewal has been arranged

## Salisbury District Hospital Library

Telephone: Salisbury (01722) 336262  extn. 4432 / 33
Out of hours answer machine in operation

# Contents

# Acknowledgements

This book would not have come into being without the support and drive of Catherine Barnes, Georgia Pinteau and Sara Chare at Oxford University Press.

The volume and series editor, Dr Chantal Simon, has been an inspiration and encouragement through the complete gestation period of this publication. In addition, Chantal was more than an active midwife in the final stages of this labour – she transformed the text and content beyond our capability with her editorial flair and wisdom

We would also like to thank Dr Ian Wright and Dr Zöe Crosby for their help reviewing this book and the authors of *The Oxford Handbook of Palliative Care* and *Oxford Handbook of General Practice* for allowing us to reproduce material, particularly Dr Hazel Everitt for material used in the chapter on non-malignant pain scenarios.

Finally we would like to thank Dr Nick Dunn for information used for the sexual health page in the palliative care section, Dr Richard Davies for information on musculoskeletal pain, Mrs Lesley Boyd for providing the back self-help exercises, Mr David Hargreaves for reviewing the sections on back pain, osteoarthritis and joint injection and Dr Helen Dunkelman for reviewing the page on lymphoedema.

All those involved in writing while working clinically, will be very aware that the real cost of such work is borne by families, and our families in Four Marks and Dungannon are no exception. We would like them to know that their patience and tolerance is appreciated.

KOR
MW

# Symbols and abbreviations

| | |
|---|---|
| ⚠ | Warning |
| ❶ | Important note |
| ☙ | Controversial point |
| ☎ | Telephone number |
| 💾 | Website |
| 📖 | Cross reference to |
| ± | With or without |
| ↑ | Increased/increasing |
| ↓ | Decreased/decreasing |
| → | Leading to |
| 1° | Primary |
| 2° | Secondary |
| ♂ | Male |
| ♀ | Female |
| ≈ | Approximately equal |
| ~ | Approximately |
| % | Percent(age) |
| ≥ | Greater than or equal to |
| ≤ | Less than or equal to |
| > | Greater than |
| < | Less than |
| +ve | Positive |
| −ve | Negative |
| ° | Degrees |
| £ | GMS contract payment available |
| C | Cochrane review |
| G | Guideline from major guideline producing body |
| N | NICE guidance |
| R | Randomized controlled trial in major journal |
| S | Systematic review in major journal |
| 5-HT | Serotonin |
| µmol/l | Micromoles per litre |

| | |
|---|---|
| AA | Attendance Allowance |
| A&E | Accident and Emergency |
| ACE | Angiotensin converting enzyme |
| AF | Atrial fibrillation |
| AIDS | Acquired immune deficiency syndrome |
| Alk phos | Alkaline phosphatase |
| AST | Aspartate amino transferase |
| bd | Twice daily |
| BJGP | British Journal of General Practice |
| BM | Blood glucose measurement on finger prick test |
| BMA | British Medical Association |
| BMD | Bone mineral density |
| BMJ | British Medical Journal |
| BNF | British National Formulary |
| BP | Blood pressure |
| bpm | Beats per minute |
| C | Centigrade |
| $Ca^{2+}$ | Calcium |
| CAM | Complementary and alternative medicine |
| CCF | Congestive cardiac failure |
| CHD | Coronary heart disease |
| cm | Centimetre(s) |
| CNS | Central nervous system |
| COC | Combined oral contraceptive pill |
| COPD | Chronic obstructive pulmonary disease |
| COX2 | Cyclo-oxygenase 2 inhibitor |
| CPN | Community psychiatric nurse |
| Cr | Creatinine |
| CRP | C-reactive protein |
| CSF | Cerebrospinal fluid |
| CSM | Committee on Safety in Medicine |
| CT | Computed tomography scan |
| CVA | Stroke |
| CVD | Cardiovascular disease |
| Cr | Creatinine |
| CXR | Chest X-ray |
| d. | Day(s) |
| DLA | Disability Living Allowance |

| DM | Diabetes mellitus |
|---|---|
| DN | District nurse |
| DoH | Department of Health |
| DTB | Drugs and Therapeutic Bulletin |
| DVLA | Driver and Vehicle Licensing Authority |
| DVT | Deep vein thrombosis |
| EC | Enteric coated |
| Echo | Echocardiogram |
| ECG | Electrocardiograph |
| e.g. | For example |
| ENT | Ear, nose and throat |
| ESR | Erythrocyte sedimentation rate |
| etc. | Et cetera |
| F | Fahrenheit |
| FBC | Full blood count |
| FH | Family history |
| g | Grams |
| GGT or γGT | Gamma glutmyl transferase |
| GI | gastrointestinal |
| GMS | General Medical Services |
| GP | General Practitioner |
| GU | Genitourinary |
| h. | Hour(s) |
| HGV | Heavy goods vehicle |
| HRT | Hormone replacement therapy |
| HSV | Herpes simplex virus |
| IBS | Irritable bowel syndrome |
| ICP | Intracranial pressure |
| IM | Intramuscular |
| INR | International normalization ratio |
| IS | Income support |
| IT | Information technology |
| IV | Intravenous |
| IVP | Intravenous pyelogram |
| JAMA | Journal of the American Medical Association |
| JSA | JobSeekers Allowance |
| JVP | Jugular venous pressure |
| $K^+$ | Potassium |

| | |
|---|---|
| kg | Kilogram(s) |
| L | Lumbar nerve root |
| LA | Local anaesthetic |
| LFTs | Liver function tests |
| LMC | Local Medical Committee |
| LMN | Lower motor neurone |
| LMWH | Low molecular weight heparin |
| LN | Lymph node |
| LOC | Loss of consciousness |
| LVF | Left ventricular failure |
| M,C&S | Microscopy, culture and sensitivities |
| m. | Metres |
| mcgm. | Micrograms |
| mg | Milligrams |
| $Mg^{2+}$ | Magnesium |
| MI | Myocardial infarct |
| min. | Minutes |
| ml | Millilitres |
| mm | Millimetres |
| mmHg | Millimetres of mercury |
| mmol/l | Millimoles per litre |
| MND | Motor neurone disease |
| mo. | Month(s) |
| MoD | Ministry of Defence |
| MRI | Magnetic resonance imaging |
| MS | Multiple sclerosis |
| MSU | Mid-stream urine |
| NEJM | New England Journal of Medicine |
| NHS | National Health Service |
| NI | Northern Ireland |
| NICE | National Institute for Clinical Excellence |
| NNT | Number needed to treat |
| nocte | At night |
| NSAID | Non-steroidal anti-inflammatory drug |
| NSF | National Service Framework |
| $O_2$ | Oxygen |
| OA | Osteoarthritis |

| od | Once daily |
|---|---|
| OT | Occupational therapy/ therapist |
| OTC | Over the counter |
| OTFC | Oral transmucosal fentanyl citrate |
| OUP | Oxford University Press |
| p. | Page number |
| PCO | Primary Care Organization |
| PE | Pulmonary embolus |
| PEG | Percutaneous endoscopic gastrostomy |
| Physio | Physiotherapy |
| PID | Pelvic inflammatory disease |
| PMH | Past medical history |
| PMR | Polymyalgia rheumatica |
| PMS | Personal Medical Services |
| po | Oral |
| $PO_4$ | Phosphate |
| PPI | Proton pump inhibitor |
| pr | Per rectum |
| prn | As needed |
| PSV | Public service vehicle |
| PU | Peptic ulceration |
| qds | Four times daily |
| RBC | Red blood cell |
| RCGP | Royal College of General Practitioners |
| RCT | Randomized controlled trial |
| s. or sec. | Second(s) |
| S | Sacral nerve root |
| SAH | Subarachnoid haemorrhage |
| s/cut | Subcutaneously |
| SI | Sacro-iliac |
| SIGN | Scottish Intercollegiate Guidelines Network |
| s/ling | Sub-lingual |
| SLR | Straight leg raise |
| SNRI | Serotonin and noradrenaline reuptake inhibitor |
| SOB | Shortness of breath |
| SR | Slow-release |
| SSRI | Selective serotonin reuptake inhibitor |
| SVC | Superior vena cava |

| TB | Tuberculosis |
|---|---|
| TCA | Tricyclic antidepressant |
| tds | Three times a day |
| TENS | Transcutaneous electrical nerve stimulation |
| TFTs | Thyroid function tests |
| TSH | Thyroid stimulating hormone |
| u. | Unit(s) |
| U&E | Urea and electrolytes |
| UC | Ulcerative colitis |
| UK | United Kingdom |
| UMN | Upper motor neurone |
| USS | Ultrasound scan |
| UTI | Urinary tract infection |
| VDU | Visual display unit |
| WHO | World Health Organization |
| wk. | Week(s) |
| y. | Year(s) |

# Chapter 1

# Assessing patients with pain symptoms in primary care

1

# What is pain?

Pain is a common symptom. We face it day after day in our work in all its different guises – from sore knees, broken bones, period pains through chronic back pain to pain from bony metastases.

Although we can't expect to have experienced all our patients' symptoms, most of us can identify at least 2–3 types of pain, and so understand that pain can mean different things at different times to different people.

It would be foolish to think that there was one simple pathway causing pain, but sometimes in our busy working lives it is easy to reach for the BNF and hope to cure-all with a small selection of 'favourite' drugs. It is important to understand not only the mechanism by which the pain is generated and possible effective treatment options, but also the symptom in its wider context in respect of the individual patient.

**Definitions of pain**: Definition depends on perspective. Here are a selection of definitions from dictionaries, patients, doctors and scientists.

- Pain is "an unpleasant feeling caused by injury or disease" or "suffering in the mind." *Oxford Mini School Dictionary*
- Pain is "what the patient says hurts"
- Pain is "an unpleasant sensory and emotional experience associated with actual or potential tissue damage or described in terms of such damage." Robert Twycross (International Association for the Study of Pain)
- Pain is "a complex physiological and emotional experience and not a simple sensation"
- Pain is "what the patient says when they want you to do something"
- Pain is "orrid!"

**Mechanism of pain:** Pain is generated by a variety of mechanisms. It is not unusual to have ≥2 mechanisms contributing to a patient's experience of pain. *Broad categories:*

**Nociceptive pain:** Pain resulting from stimulation of peripheral nerves transmitted by an undamaged nervous system. Pain impulses enter the spinal cord through the dorsal horn, where they ascend to higher centres in the brain. Usually opioid responsive.

**Neuropathic pain:** Pain arising from a damaged peripheral or central nervous system. Pain is associated with altered sensation such as burning or numbness. Neuropathic pain is usually only partially opioid responsive.

- *Peripheral pain:* Damage to the peripheral nervous system. Often associated with altered sensation around the site of nerve injury.
- *Central pain:* Damage within the central nervous system. There is usually an area of altered sensation incorporating the area of pain. Common causes include CVA or spinal cord damage.
- *Sympathetically maintained pain:* Due to sympathetic nerve injury. Essential features are pain (often burning) and sensory disorder in a vascular as opposed to a neural distribution. In patients with cancer such pain is more common in the lower limbs, and is usually associated with disease in the pelvis.

## GP Notes: Pain terminology

- **Allodynia** Pain caused by a stimulus that does not normally provoke pain
- **Analgesia** Absence of pain in response to stimulation that would normally be painful
- **Causalgia** A syndrome of sustained burning pain, allodynia and hyperpathia after a traumatic nerve lesion – often combined with vasomotor dysfunction, and later with trophic changes
- **Central pain** Pain associated with a lesion in the central nervous system (brain and spinal cord)
- **Dysaesthesia** Unpleasant abnormal sensation, which can be either spontaneous or provoked
- **Hyperaesthesia** ↑ sensitivity to stimulation
- **Hyperalgesia** ↑ response to a stimulus that is normally painful
- **Hyperpathia** Painful syndrome characterized by ↑ reaction to a stimulus – especially a repetitive stimulus – as well as ↑ threshold.
- **Neuralgia** Pain in the distribution of a nerve
- **Neuropathy** A disturbance of function or pathological change in a nerve
- **Neuropathic** Pain that is transmitted by a damaged nervous system and which is usually only partially opioid sensitive
- **Nociceptor** A receptor preferentially sensitive to a noxious stimulus or to a stimulus that would become noxious if prolonged
- **Nociceptive** Pain that is transmitted by an undamaged nervous pain system and which is usually opioid responsive.

### Figure 1.1 Picture of pain by Olan aged 10y.

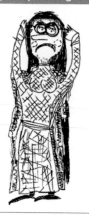

**Acute versus chronic pain:** It is critical for doctor and patient to appreciate the difference between acute and chronic pain.

**Acute pain:**
- Is a symptom of injured or diseased tissue
- Provides us with a protective reflex – we know to stop an activity when it causes pain
- Can be made worse by fear
- Subsides when the injury has finished healing.

Medical treatment for acute pain focuses on healing the underlying cause of the pain.

**Chronic pain:** Defined as pain persisting for >3–6mo. Affects ~7% of adults in the UK. There are at least two different types of chronic pain:
- Chronic pain due to an identifiable and ongoing cause
- Chronic pain with no identifiable pain generator. This type of pain does not serve any protective or other biological function.

In both cases, cause is often multidimensional – with physical, social, and psychological factors contributing to the overall impression of pain.

Treatment differs depending on the underlying cause of the pain and other factors which contribute to the sensation of pain. A multidisciplinary approach and realistic targets are essential. Abolition of pain may be impossible – 70% have ongoing pain despite analgesia. The aim of treatment is often rehabilitation with ↓ in distress/disability.

**Scientific versus holistic approach:** As clinicians, we sometimes take a scientific or holistic approach to pain assessment and management. Neither is ideal.

**The scientific clinician:** can be so specialized in synapse research that his/her model of pain control may appear simplistic and mechanistic, particularly if conveyed with the certitude that this model of pain alleviation is the only valid approach. While important advances in pain management have arisen from this model, the day-to-day experience of patients in pain in the clinical situation betrays a much more complex picture of the nature of pain.

**The holistic clinician:** in contrast, can view patients' pain with such a wide-angle holistic lens that the specifics of the patient's particular pain are ignored.

## GP Notes:

ℹ Remember that pain can be affected by a number of ever-changing parameters, only one of which is the underlying pathological process.

# Assessment of pain

*'It is more important to know what sort of person has a disease than to know what sort of disease a person has.'*
Hippocrates (460–377 BC)

## Aim to understand
- What the patient means when they complain of pain
- How the symptom is affecting this patient's life
- The patient's ideas and concerns about the symptom
- The patient's expectations
- Whether there are any antagonizing factors that can be addressed
- The mechanism by which the pain is generated and target pharmacological interventions appropriately.

Assessment is not a 'one-off' event, but an ongoing process constantly re-evaluated as more information is gathered. Assessment requires attention to the scientific processes underlying the symptom and holistic issues affecting presentation of that person's pain at this particular time.

🅘 Do not jump to conclusions or make assumptions about a patient's pain. To make an accurate assessment, listen carefully to the history – even if the clinical scenario is one you have encountered numerous times before.

**Assessment questions:** There are many approaches to assessing pain. The specifics of each scheme are not crucial, but it is important that the scheme used has a logical outline that works for the individual clinician. A simple mnemonic approach is detailed opposite (Figure 1.2).

## Practical details of pain assessment consultation:
- Seek to establish a relationship with the patient
- Is the patient currently in distress due to pain? If so, try to make the patient more comfortable before carrying out a full assessment
- Maintain eye-to-eye level contact
- Give a clear introduction
- Avoid over-familiarity and patronizing the patient
- Explain what you plan to do
- Summarize back to the patient: 'Have I heard things correctly…'
- Use language and terms appropriate to the patient.

## Pain history principles:
- Encourage the patient to do most of the talking
- Begin with 'wide-angle' open questions before clarifying and focusing with more specific ones
- Watch the patient for clues regarding pain
- Assess the severity of pain as objectively as possible
- Assess the degree to which the pain is affecting the patients function/daily activities.

**Always examine the patient…** The cause of the problem may be clear to you from history alone but **DON'T** underestimate the therapeutic value to the patient of being examined. It may seem outdated to believe 'laying on of hands' has in itself a value, but it has an importance out of proportion to the clinical information it yields.

## Figure 1.2 Points to consider when taking a history of pain

**S** **Site of pain**: Where? Any radiation? Numbness where pain felt? Pattern of joint/muscle involvement?

**O** **Onset**: When did it start? How did it start? What started it? Change over time? History of injury?

**C** **Character of pain**: Type of pain – burning, shooting, stabbing, dull etc., pattern of pain e.g. colicky, constant etc.

**R** **Radiation**: Does the pain go anywhere else?

**A** **Associated features** : Are there any skin or joint changes e.g. bruising redness or swelling?

**T** **Timing/pattern**: Is it worse at any time of day? Is it associated with any particular activities? e.g. movement, urination, eating, passing stool, coughing?

**E** **Exacerbating and relieving factors**

**S** **Severity**: Record especially if the pain is chronic and you want to measure change over time. Consider a patient diary. Ask about:
- Pain intensity e.g. none–mild–moderate–severe; rank on a 1–10 scale.
- Record interference with sleep or usual activities
- Pain relief e.g. none–slight–moderate–good–complete.

#### GP Notes:

⚠ Remember that as you are assessing patients, they are assessing you.

**Pain assessment tools:** Symptom monitoring by patients using pain diaries and/or pain scales (Figure 1.3) can be used to enhance understanding of symptoms and improve assessment of the effectiveness of management strategies. Used appropriately, such evaluation tools provide a quantifiable measure which both patient and healthcare professional can use to chart the effectiveness of pain-reducing interventions. However, for those patients who may ruminate about their 'pain scores', the use of such a method of assessment exacerbates pain and pain awareness.

**Secondary effects of pain:** Experience of pain can induce/antagonize other clinical and psychosocial problems. These secondary effects constantly affect the patient's experience of pain. Experience of pain can:

- Induce depression
- Exacerbate anxiety
- Interfere with social performance
- Negatively impact on physical capability
- Prevent a patient working
- Decrease income
- Encourage isolation
- Impair the quality of relationships and sexuality
- Create family disharmony and stress
- Challenge existential beliefs

### Elderly patients and patients with difficulty communicating:

The high prevalence of pain in the elderly population is now well recognized. One study showed 40–80% of elderly people in institutions are in pain. Many patients suffering from dementia receive no pain relief at all, despite the presence of concomitant, potentially painful illnesses. The reason for this lies in the difficulty in assessing those with communication difficulties. Additionally, the elderly often minimize their pain making it even more difficult to evaluate.

**Methods of evaluation:** Unusual behaviour and its return to normal with adequate analgesia, may be the only confirmation of pain in patients with communication difficulties. Examples include:

*Verbal expression* e.g.
- Crying when touched
- Shouting
- Becoming very quiet
- Swearing
- Grunting
- Talking without making sense

*Behavioural expression* e.g.
- Jumping on touch
- Hand pointing to body area
- Increasing confusion
- Rocking/shaking
- Not eating
- Staying in bed/chair
- Grumpy mood

*Facial expression* e.g.
- Grimacing/wincing
- Closing eyes
- Worried expression
- Withdrawn/no expression

*Physical expression* e.g.
- Cold
- Pale
- Clammmy
- Change in 'colour'
- Change in vital signs if acute pain (e.g. BP, pulse)

8

**Figure 1.3 Simple visual analogue pain scale**

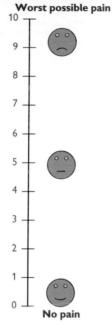

**Worst possible pain**

10

9

8

7

6

5

4

3

2

1

0

**No pain**

Ask the patient to mark a point on the line that represents their current pain level – where 10 is the worst pain they have ever experienced and 0 is 'no pain at all'.

# Chapter 2

# Chronic pain relief

# Chronic pain control

In the UK, 7% of adults have chronic pain. Pain is always subjective so there is little point in arguing whether a patient has pain or not. Management of pain must include a thought for 'what exactly is pain?' and 'what exactly is it for this patient?' Chronic pain is usually multifactorial and effective management represents a partnership between the patient and/or carers and doctor (Figure 2.1).

**Assessment:** 📖 p.6–9.

## Goals of pain management:
- Set realistic targets
- Abolition of pain may be impossible – 70% of patients have pain despite analgesia
- If analgesia is not helping – stop it
- The aim is often rehabilitation to ↓ distress/disability.

**Strategies for pain management:** A multidisciplinary approach is essential. *Consider:*
- *Prevention:* e.g. wrist splints for carpal tunnel syndrome; analgesia prior to minor surgery
- *Removal of cause:* Treat medical causes of pain e.g. infection, ↓ blood sugar (diabetic neuropathy). Refer surgical causes for surgery if appropriate e.g. hip osteoarthritis – joint replacement.
- *Pain-relieving drugs:* Start with a single drug at low dose and step up dose or add another drug as needed – 📖 p.101. Especially in situations of acute pain, step down treatment if pain diminishes.
- *Physical therapies:* Acupuncture, physiotherapy or TENS
- *Nerve blocks:* Consider referral for epidural (low back pain), local nerve block or sympathectomy (e.g. vascular rest pain)
- *Modification of emotional response:* Psychotropic drugs e.g. anxiolytics, antidepressants
- *Modification of behavioural response:* e.g. back pain – consider referral to a back rehabilitation scheme.

**Referral:** If unable to remove cause and unable to achieve adequate pain relief, consider referral to a specialist pain-control clinic or for palliative care (whichever is more appropriate).

## Address patient concerns:
Common concerns include:
- Finding and using health services and other community resources
- Knowing how to recognize/respond to changes in a chronic disease
- Dealing with problems and emergencies
- Making decisions about when to seek medical help
- Using medicines and treatments effectively
- Managing stress and depression that accompany a chronic illness
- Coping with fatigue, pain, and sleep problems
- Getting enough exercise and maintaining good nutrition
- Working with the doctor(s) and other care providers
- Talking about the illness with family and friends
- Managing work, family, and social activities.

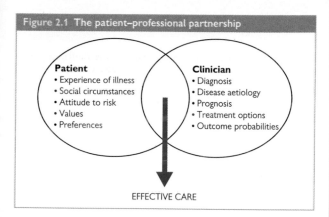

Figure 2.1 The patient–professional partnership

**Patient**
- Experience of illness
- Social circumstances
- Attitude to risk
- Values
- Preferences

**Clinician**
- Diagnosis
- Disease aetiology
- Prognosis
- Treatment options
- Outcome probabilities

EFFECTIVE CARE

**GP Notes:**

⚠ In management of chronic pain, prescription of analgesic medication will rarely be the sole therapeutic tool.

**Expert patient schemes:** 6wk. courses led by an 'expert patient' rather than health professional. Aim to train people with long-term chronic conditions e.g. arthritis to 'self-manage' their condition more effectively on a day-to-day basis. Topics covered are generic not disease specific e.g. medicines management. Each week participants attend a $2\frac{1}{2}$ h. session in groups of ~13. Also available on-line.

**Advice for patients: Useful contacts**

**Action on pain** ☎ 0845 603 1593 🖳 www.action-on-pain.co.uk
**Pain concern** ☎ 01620 822 572 🖳 www.painconcern.org.uk
**Pain Association of Scotland** ☎ 0800 783 6059
🖳 www.painassociation.com

**Further information:**

British Pain Society 🖳 www.britishpainsociety.org
Moore et al. *Bandolier's Little Book of Pain.* OUP 2003, ISBN: 0192632477
The Oxford Pain Internet Site 🖳 www.jr2.ox.ac.uk/bandolier/booth/painpag
Expert Patient Programme 🖳 www.expertpatients.nhs.uk

# The analgesic ladder

Most pain can be managed using a step-by-step approach (Figure 2.2).

## Step 1: Non-opioid:

- Start treatment with paracetamol. Stress the need for REGULAR dosage. Adult dose is 1g every 4–6h. regularly (maximum daily dose 4g).
- If this is not adequate in 24 h., either try a NSAID e.g. ibuprofen 400mg tds (if appropriate) alone or in combination with paracetamol, or proceed to step 2.

## Step 2: Weak opioid + non-opioid:

- Start treatment with a combined preparation of paracetamol with codeine or dihydrocodeine. Combining 2 analgesics with different mechanisms of action enables better pain control than using either drug alone at that dose
- Combinations have ↓ dose-related side effects but the range of side effects is ↑ (additive effects of 2 drugs)
- Combinations using 30mg of codeine (e.g. Solpadol®) are more effective than paracetamol alone but it is cheaper and more flexible if constituents are prescribed separately e.g. 'paracetamol 500mg/codeine 30mg'
- Advise patients to take tablets regularly and not to assess efficacy after only a couple of doses.

⊘ There is no proven additional analgesic benefit from preparations that contain paracetamol + 8mg codeine, as opposed to paracetamol alone.

## Step 3: Strong opioid + non-opioid:

- Use immediate-release morphine tablets or morphine solution. 2 tablets of co-codamol contain 60mg of codeine which is equi-analgesic to ~6mg of oral morphine. If changing to morphine, use a minimum dose of 5mg (6mg is hard to prescribe)
- Chronic pain may be only partially opioid sensitive. Give for a 2wk. trial and only continue if of proven benefit. Worries of tolerance/addiction are unfounded for patients with true opioid-sensitive pain. If the pain seems responsive to opioids and there are no undue side effects, ↑ the dose upwards by 30–50% every 24h. until pain is controlled – 📖 p.100.

⚠ Take care if the patient is elderly or in renal failure – consider starting with a ↓ dose of morphine – 📖 p.44.

**Addition of co-analgesics and adjuvant drugs:** In combination with analgesics, can enhance pain control. Examples include:

- *Antidepressants* – in low dose for nerve pain and sleep disturbance associated with pain; in larger doses for secondary depression
- *Anticonvulsants* – neuropathic pain
- *Corticosteroids* – pain due to oedema
- *Muscle relaxants* – muscle cramp pain
- *Antispasmodics* – bowel colic
- *Antibiotics* – infection pain
- *Night sedative* – when lack of sleep is lowering pain threshold
- *Anxiolytic* – when anxiety is making pain worse (relaxation exercises may also help in these circumstances).

## Figure 2.2 World Health Organization (WHO) analgesics ladder[1] (reproduced with permission)

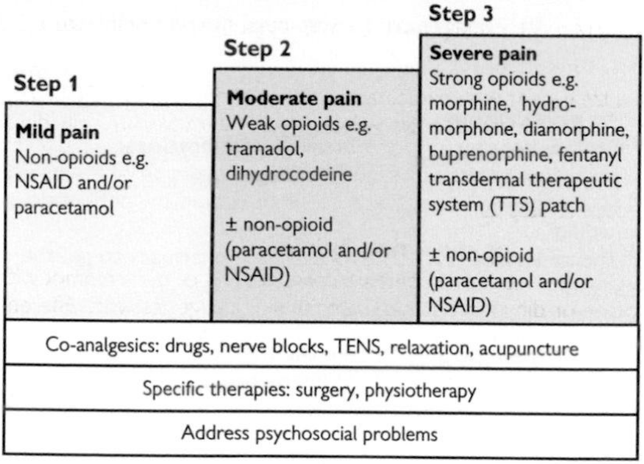

| Step 1 | Step 2 | Step 3 |
|---|---|---|
| **Mild pain**<br>Non-opioids e.g. NSAID and/or paracetamol | **Moderate pain**<br>Weak opioids e.g. tramadol, dihydrocodeine<br><br>± non-opioid (paracetamol and/or NSAID) | **Severe pain**<br>Strong opioids e.g. morphine, hydro-morphone, diamorphine, buprenorphine, fentanyl transdermal therapeutic system (TTS) patch<br><br>± non-opioid (paracetamol and/or NSAID) |

Co-analgesics: drugs, nerve blocks, TENS, relaxation, acupuncture

Specific therapies: surgery, physiotherapy

Address psychosocial problems

**GP Notes:**

⚠ Be aware of 2° gain from pain if symptoms seem out of proportion (outstanding compensation claims are a significant negative factor in the success of pain management).

## Further information:

**British Pain Society** 🖥 www.britishpainsociety.org
- Recommendations for the appropriate use of opioids for persistent non-cancer pain (2005)
- A practical guide to the provision of chronic pain services for adults in primary care (2004).

1 World Health Organization (1996). Cancer Pain Relief: With a Guide to Opioid Availability. 2nd edition. Geneva: WHO.

# Practical considerations

*'I've never had a problem with drugs. I've had problems with the police.'*

Keith Richards

## Prior to prescribing
### 1. Will the patient be able to obtain the medications?
- Will the drugs prescribed require a special order from the pharmacy and take a few days to arrive? If so, what should the patient do meanwhile?
- Will the patient/carer be able to go to the pharmacy to get the medication?
- Does the local pharmacy deliver?

### 2. Will the patient be able to take the medication safely?
- Does the patient understand the instructions?
- Would writing the instructions help?
- Would a dosette box help?
- Have you prescribed enough medication to last until you next see the patient?
- Might the medication run out over the weekend? If so, does the patient/carer know what to do if supplies run out?
- Have you prescribed any additional medication needed e.g. a laxative with opioids?
- Have you advised patient/carer what to do with any previous unused medicines?

### 3. Follow up?
- Does the patient know what to do if side effects develop?
- Does the patient know what to do in an emergency?
- Have you left some way of communicating your plans for other health care professionals in the team e.g. district nurse, emergency visiting doctor?
- Have you arranged to review the situation and does the patient know this?

## If medication doesn't work
*'I'm in so much pain – those tablets you gave me are not working at all.'*

Sound familiar? **Before** you reach for your prescription pad, ask yourself:
- Is the diagnosis correct?
- Does the clinical scenario need to be re-evaluated?
- Has some other pathological process supervened?
- Is re-examination warranted?
- Could the pain be originating from an alternative pathological process?
- Is my method of evaluating the pain sound?
- Do I have a way of assessing when the pain is 'better' or 'worse?'
- Have I explored how the pain affects functioning?
- Has something happened to alter the patient's perception of pain?
- Has something happened to cause the emotional distress?
- Is the patient actually taking the medication?
- Has the correct dose of analgesia been prescribed for an adequate trial period?

## GP Notes:

If analgesia is not working, could the pain be opioid resistant?

### Pseudo-opioid-resistant pain

- Underdosing
- Poor alimentary absorption of opioid (rare, except where there is an ileostomy)
- Poor alimentary intake because of vomiting

### Partially opioid-sensitive pain

- Bone pain
- Raised intracranial pressure
- Neuropathic pain
- Activity-related pain

### Opioid-resistant pain

- Muscle spasm
- Abdominal cramps
- Spiritual pain – patients with chronic unremitting pain from a deteriorating condition are particularly at risk of spiritual pain. Referral for psychological/spiritual support is important, and/or use of a complementary therapy.

# Concordance

When medication is reported as ineffective it is common to find the patient has not been taking the drug in the manner it that was prescribed. 'Paracetamol doesn't help' *to the doctor* means '2 tablets every 4 hours are ineffective' but *to the patient* may mean '2 tablets in the morning does not keep me pain free all day.'

**Concordance:** is a process of prescribing and medicine-taking based on partnership. Patient concordance (or, rather, lack of it) is a major challenge in general practice. For drugs to be optimally effective they must be taken as directed by the prescriber. Concordance sufficient to attain therapeutic objectives occurs ~ $^1/_2$ of the time:
- 1:6 patients take medication exactly as directed
- 1:3 take medication as directed 80–90% of the time
- 1:3 take medication as directed 40–80% of the time
- The remaining 16–17% take medication as directed <40% of the time
- 20% of prescriptions are never 'cashed'.

## Causes of non-concordance

**Patient beliefs:** Strongest predictor of compliance – how natural a medicine is seen to be, the dangers of addiction and dependence, and the belief that constant use may lead to ↓ efficacy influence compliance.

**Lifestyle choices:**
- Unpleasant side effects – especially if not pre-warned
- Inconvenience e.g. multiple daily dosage regimens – though there is little difference between od and bd dosage
- No perceived benefit
- Hearsay evidence of adverse effects 'Auntie Joan took those tablets and she was dead within a week'.

**Information:** Instructions not understood, not passed on to carers or poor understanding of the condition/treatment.

**Practical reasons:** Forgetfulness; inability to open containers.

**Poor patient–professional relationship:**
- There is a link between patient satisfaction with a consultation and subsequent concordance
- Inappropriate prescribing
- Mistakes in administration/dispensing.

**Improving concordance:** ~70% of patients want to be more involved in decisions about treatment. Doctors underestimate the degree to which they instruct and overestimate the degree to which they consult and elicit their patients' views. The doctor's task is, by negotiation, to help patients choose the best way to manage their problem. Patients are more likely to be motivated to take medicines as prescribed when they:
- Understand and accept the diagnosis
- Agree with the treatment proposed
- Have had their concerns about the medicines specifically and seriously addressed.

## GP Notes: Ways to improve concordance

- Use simple language and avoid medical terms
- Discuss reasons for treatment and consequences of not treating the condition, ensuring information is tailored, clear, accurate, accessible, and sufficiently detailed
- Seek a patient's view on their condition
- Agree a course of action before prescribing
- Explain what the drug is, its function and (if known and not too complex) its mechanism of action
- Keep the drug regimen as simple as possible – od or bd dosing is preferable especially long-term
- Ensure 12 hourly medication is taken 12-hourly and not simply 2×/d. to ensure consistent pain relief over 24 hours
- Seek the patient's views on how they will manage the regimen within their daily schedule and try to tie it in with daily routine (e.g. take one tablet in the morning when you get up)
- Discuss possible side effects – especially common or unpleasant side effects
- Give clear verbal instructions and reinforce with written instructions if it is a complex regimen, the patient is elderly, or understanding of the patient is in doubt
- Deal with any questions the patient has
- Repeat information yourself and also ask patients to repeat information back to you to reinforce information
- If necessary, arrange a review within a short time of starting a medicine to discuss progress or queries, or arrange follow up by another member of the primary health care team (e.g. asthma nurse to check inhaler technique 2–3wk. after starting inhaler)
- Address further patient questions and practical difficulties at follow up
- Monitor repeat prescriptions.

**Further information:**

NICE Medicines adherence involving patients in decisions about prescribed medicines and supporting adherence (2009) 📖 www.nice.org.uk

# Paracetamol and non-steroidal anti-inflammatory drugs (NSAIDs)

**Paracetamol:** *BNF 4.7.1*
- As effective a painkiller as ibuprofen
- No anti-inflammatory effect but potent antipyretic
- Drug of choice in osteoarthritis where inflammation is absent
- Side effects are rare
- Dosage 1g qds
- Overdose (>4g/24h.) can be fatal causing hepatic damage sometimes not apparent for 4–6d
- Inadvertent overdose is easy due to presence of paracetamol in most over-the-counter cold preparations – refer to A&E.

**Non-steroidal anti-inflammatories (NSAIDs):** *BNF 10.1.1* Table 2.1
- Anti-inflammatory, analgesic, antipyretic
- Start at the lowest recommended dose and don't use >1 NSAID concurrently
- 60% of patients respond to any NSAID – for those who don't, another may work.

*GI side effects:* Common (50%) including GI bleeds ($^1/_4$ of GI bleeds in the UK). ↑ with age. Risks are dose related and vary between drugs.
- For the elderly, those on steroids or with past history of a drug-induced GI bleed or indigestion, protect the stomach with misoprostol or a proton pump inhibitor (PPI)
- Selective inhibitors of cyclo-oxygenase-2 (COX2) are as with less GI side effects effective as NSAIDs as but should not be given to any patient with pre-existing or high risk of cardio- or cerebrovascular disease.

*Other side effects:*
- Hypersensitivity reactions – 5–10% of asthmatics develop bronchospasm
- Fluid retention – relative contraindication in patients with ↑BP/cardiac failure
- Renal failure – rare – more common in patients with pre-existing renal disease
- Hepatic impairment – particularly with diclofenac.

🛇 COX2 inhibitors:
- Have NO effect on platelet aggregation
- Have no benefit over non-selective NSAIDs if used in patients on continuous low-dose aspirin
- Combining a COX2 inhibitor with PPI/misoprostol does NOT give extra stomach protection.

**Topical NSAIDs:** Of proven benefit for acute and chronic conditions[s] and can be as effective as oral preparations. They have a lower incidence of GI and other side effects, though these still occur.

**Combination analgesics:** 📖 p.14.

| Table 2.1 Commonly used NSAIDs *(BNF 10.1.1)* | | |
|---|---|---|
| **Drug** | **Dosage** | **Features** |
| Ibuprofen | 1.2–1.8g/d. in 3–4 divided doses | Fewer side effects than other NSAIDs. Anti-inflammatory properties are weaker. Do not use if inflammation is prominent e.g. gout. |
| Naproxen | 0.5–1g/d. in 1–2 divided doses | Good efficacy with a low incidence of side-effects. |
| Diclofenac | 75–150mg/d. in 1–2 divided doses | |
| Meloxicam | 7.5–15mg od | Selective COX2 inhibitors. As effective as non-selective NSAIDs and share side effects but risk of serious upper GI events is lower. Only use if at low risk of cerebro- or cardiovascular disease and high risk of GI side effects. |
| Celecoxib | 200mg od or bd | |

### GP Notes:

#### Use of NSAIDs:

- All NSAIDs are associated with GI toxicity – risk is ↑ in the elderly
- Use lower-risk NSAIDs e.g. ibuprofen as first-line treatment
- Start at the lowest recommended dose
- Do not use >1 oral NSAID at a time
- Remember that *all* NSAIDs are contraindicated in patients with active peptic ulceration. Non-selective NSAIDs are contraindicated in patients with a history of peptic ulceration.

🔴 Combination of a NSAID and low-dose aspirin may ↑ risk of GI side effects: only use this combination if absolutely necessary and if the patient is monitored closely.

**COX2 inhibitors:** Due to concerns about cardiovascular safety, *only* use COX2 inhibitors in preference to standard NSAIDs when specifically indicated (i.e. for patients at high risk of developing gastro-duodenal ulcer, perforation, or bleeding) and after an assessment of cardiovascular risk. Switch patients receiving a COX2 inhibitor who have ischaemic heart disease or cerebrovascular disease to alternative treatment.

### Further information:

**Bandolier** Topical NSAIDs (2003)
🖥 www.jr2.ox.ac.uk/bandolier/band110/b110-6.html

# Weak opioids

**Codeine:** The most commonly used weak opioid in the UK. Dose is 30–60mg every 4h. to a maximum of 240mg/24h. Analgesic effect is increased by regular ingestion.

**Equipotence with morphine:** 60mg of codeine 4x/d. totals 240mg codeine in 24h. 10mg of codeine is equipotent to 1mg of morphine so the equivalent morphine dose would be 24mg/24h.

**Side effects:** The most common side effects include nausea, vomiting, constipation, and drowsiness (📖 p.34). Codeine is effective for the relief of mild to moderate pain but is too constipating for long-term use. Always consider prescribing a laxative e.g. bisacodyl 1–2 tablets nocte with codeine to prevent constipation.

### Reasons for decreased effectiveness:
- 5–10% of Caucasians have the CYP2D6 genotype. They lack a hepatic enzyme necessary to convert codeine to morphine and will obtain less analgesia when taking codeine-containing analgesics
- Effects of codeine are reduced by concurrent use of:
  - Antipsychotics e.g. chlorpromazine, haloperidol, levomepromazine
  - Metoclopramide
  - Tricyclic antidepressants e.g. amitriptyline.

**Dihydrocodeine:** has analgesic efficacy and side effect profile similar to that of codeine. The dose of dihydrocodeine by mouth is 30–60mg every 4h. A 40–mg tablet is now also available.

**Tramadol:** is a synthetic analogue of codeine. It is not a controlled drug. Dose range 50mg bd, increasing to a maximum of 400mg/24h. Produces analgesia by two mechanisms:
- An opioid effect
- An enhancement of serotonergic and adrenergic pathways.

**Preparations:** Table 2.2

**Side effects:** 📖 p.34

### Advantages over codeine and dihydrocodeine
- Rapid absorption of oral doses – analgesia in <1h.–peaks at 1–2h
- Metabolized in the liver – safer for the elderly and those with renal failure
- Fewer typical opioid side effects (notably, ↓ respiratory depression, constipation, and addiction potential)
- May have a significant effect on neuropathic pain.

### Disadvantages
- Psychiatric reactions have been reported
- Nausea and vomiting can be a problem with high doses.

**Fentanyl and buprenorphine:** Buprenorphine is considered by some to be a weak opioid but only at low dosage. Fentanyl is a strong opioid but its delivery system influences intensity of action. In some circumstances it acts like a weak opioid 📖 pp.29 and 32.

**Compound analgesics:** 📖 p.23

## Table 2.2 Weak opioid preparations (BNF 4.7.2)

| Drug | Preparations |
|------|-------------|
| Codeine | *Syrup* – available as codeine phosphate 25mg/5ml<br>*Immediate-release tablets* – available as codeine phosphate 15, 30 and 60mg tablets<br>*Injection* – codeine phosphate 60mg/ml |
| Dihydrocodeine | *Oral solution* – available as dihydrocodeine tartrate 10mg/5ml<br>*Immediate-release tablets* – dihydrocodeine tartrate 30mg and 40mg (DF-118 Forte®)<br>*Modified-release* (bd administration) – dihydrocodeine tartrate 60, 90 and 120mg tablets (DHC Continus®)<br>*Injection* – dihydrocodeine tartrate 50mg/ml |
| Tramadol | *Immediate release* – available as 50mg capsules, 50mg soluble tablets, 50mg orodispersible tablets, and 50 and 100mg effervescent sachets<br>*Modified-release preparations:*<br>*bd dosage* – available as 50, 100, 150 and 200mg tablets and capsules<br>*od dosage* – available as 150, 200, 300 and 400mg capsules<br>*In combination with paracetamol:* 37.5mg tramadol and 325mg paracetamol tablets<br>*Injection* |

# Morphine

Morphine is the strong opioid of first choice for moderate to severe pain in both malignant and non-malignant conditions.

🚹 BNF recommends regular use of using strong opioids in non-malignant conditions should be supervised by a specialist.

## Starting a patient on morphine

**Paperwork:** To protect patients and doctors when starting a patient on morphine, regardless of whether the underlying disease is malignant or non-malignant documentation is important. *Document:*

- Indication for starting opioids
- Discussion of implications of using opioids, including implications for driving, interactions with alcohol etc.
- Proposed duration of opioid therapy and plan for monitoring
- Laxatives and antiemetics prescribed to counteract side effects

**Preparations available:** Table 2.3

**Initial dosage:** Start with immediate-release morphine liquid or tablets, depending on patient preference. A 4-hourly dose of morphine gives greatest flexibility for initial dose titration and causes fewer side effects than longer-acting preparations. Give clear instructions. Initial dosage:

- *Adults not pain-controlled with regular weak opioids* (e.g. co-codamol 500/30, 2 tablets qds) – 5–10mg oral morphine every 4h.
- *Elderly, cachectic, or not taking regular weak opioids* – 2.5–5mg morphine every 4h.
- *Very elderly and frail* – 2.5mg of morphine every 4h.

**Prevention of adverse effects:** 📖 p.34

- Always prescribe a laxative concurrently (e.g. docusate, bisacodyl).
- >1:3 patients develop nausea on starting opioids – prescribe a regular antiemetic e.g. haloperidol 1.5mg nocte. Opioid-induced nausea wears off in <2wk., so antiemetics can be converted to 'PRN' after 2wk.
- Explain that any drowsiness will usually wear off after a few days. Advise patients not to drive for at least 1wk. after starting morphine or after any increase in dose. Patients should also avoid driving after this time if drowsiness persists (📖 p.34).

**Breakthrough pain:** Defined as pain of rapid onset, moderate/severe intensity, and short duration which may be precipitated by activity but can occur spontaneously. *Management:*

- Ensure access to immediate-release morphine for breakthrough pain. Give the same dose as the 4-hourly dose (or $^1/_6$ of the total daily dose of background medication) as an additional dose.
- If pain starts to occur regularly before the next dose of analgesia is due, increase the regular *background dose*.

**Titration of dose:** Increase the dose as needed by increments of ~25–50% daily until pain is controlled or side effects prevent further increase. There is no 'maximum' daily allowance. e.g.
5→10→15→20→30→40→60→80→100→130→160→200mg

🚹 Very few patients require more than 600mg daily.

## Table 2.3 Morphine preparations *(BNF 4.7.2)*

| Drug | Preparations |
|---|---|
| *Morphine solution* | State dose of morphine to be dissolved in 5ml of chloroform water e.g. 5mg/5ml. If dose is >13mg/5ml the preparation becomes a controlled drug (p.218).<br>*Oramorph®* – 10, 30 or 100mg/5ml. |
| *Morphine sulphate immediate-release tablets* | 10, 20, or 50mg tablets. |
| *Morphine sulphate modified-release preparations* | *bd dosage:* e.g. MST Continus® – available in 5, 10, 15, 30, 60, 100, and 200mg tablets and as oral suspension.<br>*od dosage:* e.g. MXL® = available in 30, 60, 90, 120, 150 and 200mg tablets. Can open capsule and sprinkle contents on soft, cold food or swallow whole. |
| *Morphine suppositories* | Morphine sulphate or hydrochloride. 10, 15, 20, and 30mg suppositories are available. |
| *Morphine injection* | Morphine sulphate 10,15, 20, and 30mg/ml. |

## Further information:

**DTB** Opioid analgesics for cancer pain in primary care. (2005).
**British Pain Society** Recommendations for the appropriate use of opioids in persistant non-cancer pain (2005)
🖳 www.britishpainsociety.org

**Maintenance:** Once pain is controlled, consider using a long-acting preparation of equivalent dosage (e.g MST® bd or MXL® od). Calculate the total daily dose of morphine by adding together the 4-hourly doses. If using a bd long-acting regimen, halve the total to give the bd dosage.

*Example:* For patients taking 10mg of oral morphine 4 hourly, the total morphine dose is 60mg/d. = 30mg of slow-release morphine bd.

**Breakthrough pain:** If the patient experiences breakthrough pain, give additional immediate-release morphine. The dose should be equivalent to the 4-hourly dose the patient is currently taking (or $1/6$ of the total daily dose of background medication).

*Example:* If a patient taking 60mg of MST® bd experiences break-through pain, the total dose of morphine is 120mg in 24h. and the 4-hourly dose is 20mg morphine (120÷6) – so give an additional 20mg of immediate-release morphine for the pain.

**Increasing dose:** If dose ↑ is necessary, use 25–50% increments. ↑ dose rather than frequency as the medications are intended for od or bd dosing.

**Injectable morphine:** Morphine is available in injectable form, and though not as readily dissolved as diamorphine, is widely used in syringe drivers and for subcutaneous injections.

**Conversion of oral to injectable morphine:** 📖 p.27 (quick conversion opposite)

**Syringe drivers:** 📖 pp.36–9

**Incident pain:** Type of breakthrough pain caused by a particular activity e.g. getting dressed, washed. Because the pain is localized to a particular event and time in the day, increasing the total analgesic dose to prevent it is likely to cause side effects as patients will not need that level of analgesia at other points in the day. Consider:
- Avoiding precipitating activities (if possible)
- Predicting pain and giving analgesia 20min. prior to activity e.g. prior to changing dressings or movement. Suitable preparations include:
  - NSAID e.g. diclofenac
  - Immediate-release oral morphine or other opioid according to background analgesia at 50–100% of the background 4-hourly dose
  - Oral transmucosal or buccal fentanyl
  - Lorazepam 0.5mg sublingually to allay anxiety

### Side effects and toxicity: 📖 p.34

**Subacute overdosage:** Slowly progressive somnolence and respiratory depression – common in patients with renal failure. Withhold morphine for 1–2 doses then reintroduce at 25% lower dose.

**Conversion to other opioids:** 📖 p.27 (quick conversion opposite).

## GP Notes:

### Troubleshooting

- Continuing pain and frequent prn doses – ↑ regular dose
- Persisting side effects (drowsiness, jerking, vomiting, confusion) – ↓ regular dose
- Considerable pain despite marked side effects – use alternative drug

### Quick conversions

| From | To | Conversion | Example |
|------|-----|-----------|---------|
| Oral morphine (total dose) | s/cut diamorphine | ÷ by 3 | 60 ÷ 3 = 20mg diamorphine by syringe driver over 24h. |
| e.g. 10mg morphine 4-hourly = 60mg oral morphine in 24h | s/cut morphine | ÷ by 2 | 60 ÷ 2 = 30mg morphine by syringe driver over 24h. |
| | oral oxycodone | ÷ by 2 | 60 ÷ 2 = 30mg oral oxycodone in divided doses over 24h. |
| | oral hydromorphone | ÷ by 7.5 | 60 ÷ 7.5 = (60 × 2) ÷ 15 = 8mg hydromorphone in divided doses over 24h. |

ⓘ If total 24h. dose is equivalent to 360mg morphine or more – seek specialist advice.

# Alternative strong opioids

An increasing number of alternative opioids are now available (Table 2.4). It is safer to know a few strong opioids well, and build up confidence in their use, than to be acquainted with a wide range of drugs but unfamiliar with their side-effect profiles.

Few strong opioids other than morphine have the range of doses and preparations needed for routine use for chronic pain in the community.

## Reasons to choose/switch to an alternative strong opioid:
- Choice – morphine is unacceptable for some patients
- Unacceptable side effects
- Renal failure
- Patient reluctant or unable to take oral medication regularly.

## Diamorphine (heroin):
- Powerful opioid analgesic – causes less nausea/hypotension than morphine.
- Greater solubility allows effective doses to be injected in smaller volumes – which is important in the emaciated patient.
- Increase dose by 25–50% increments as for oral morphine.
- Use 50–100% of the equivalent 4-hourly dose for breakthrough pain e.g. for a patient on 180mg diamorphine/24h. through a syringe driver, 4-hourly equivalent dose is $180 \div 6 = 30$mg, so breakthrough dose is 15–30mg subcutaneously.

**Indications for switching to a syringe driver:** 📖 p.36

**Conversion of oral morphine to diamorphine:** 📖 p.29 (quick conversion opposite)

> ⚠ Diamorphine has been the injectable drug-of-choice in the UK. Alternatives include soluble morphine or oxycodone.

**Pethidine:** prompt but short-lasting analgesia; less constipating than morphine, but even in high doses is a less potent analgesic. It is not suitable for severe continuing pain due to accumulation of toxic metabolites but is frequently used in the community in injectable form for acute pain relief and/or obstetric pain.

**Methadone:** is less sedating than morphine and acts for longer periods. It is difficult to use safely in the community because of its unpredictably long half-life causing ↑ risk of accumulation and opioid overdosage. Only use under consultant supervision.

**Hydromorphone and oxycodone:** both have efficacy and side-effect profiles similar to that of morphine and are used primarily for control of pain in palliative care. There is little to choose between them, but oxycodone is often chosen in preference because:
- A liquid immediate-release and injectable form are available in the UK
- Doses are simpler to calculate
- There is less variation in the reported equianalgesic ratios.

**Conversion of oral morphine to hydromorphone and oxycodone:** 📖 p.30 (quick conversion opposite)

## Table 2.4 Other strong opioid preparations *(BNF 4.7.2)*

| Drug | Preparations |
|---|---|
| Diamorphine | Available as 10mg tablets or injection (5, 10, 30, 100 and 500mg ampoules) |
| Hydromorphone | *Immediate-release preparation* – available as 1.3 and 2.6mg capsules which can be swallowed whole or opened and contents sprinkled on soft, cold food.<br>*Modified-release (bd dosage)* – available as 2, 4, 8, 16, and 24mg capsules. |
| Oxycodone | *Immediate-release capsules* – available as 5, 10, and 20mg capsules<br>*Oral solution* – available as 5mg/5ml and 10mg/ml strengths.<br>*Modified-release (bd dosage)* – available as 5, 10, 20, 40, and 80mg tablets.<br>*Injection* – 10mg/ml × 1ml or 2ml ampoules |
| Fentanyl | *Transdermal patches:* delivering 25, 50, 75, or 100mcgm/h. for 72h. a 12mcgm/h. patch is also available for titration between doses.<br>Different buccal and sublingual preparations are now available.<br>*Lozenges:* 200, 400, 600, and 800mcgm, and 1.2 and 1.6mg doses are available. Repeat if pain not relieved in 15min. No more than 2 dose units for each pain episode and 4 dose units/d.<br>*Injection* – 50mcgm/ml × 2ml or 10ml ampoules |
| Buprenorphine | *Sublingual (Temgesic®):* available as 200 or 400mcgm tablets.<br>*Transdermal patches:* delivering 35, 52.5, or 70mcgm/h. for 72h.<br>*Injection* – 300mcgm/ml × 1ml ampoules |

29

## GP Notes: Quick conversions

| From | To | Conversion | Example |
|---|---|---|---|
| Oral morphine (total dose)<br>e.g. 10mg morphine 4-hourly = 60mg oral morphine in 24h. | s/cut diamorphine | ÷ by 3 | 60 ÷ 3 = 20mg diamorphine by syringe driver over 24h. |
| | oral oxycodone | ÷ by 2 | 60 ÷ 2 = 30mg oral oxycodone in divided doses over 24h. |
| | oral hydro-morphone | ÷ by 7.5 | 60 ÷ 7.5 = (60 × 2) ÷ 15 = 8mg hydromorphone in divided doses over 24h. |
| S/cut diamorphine | s/cut oxycodone | × 0.75 or 1 up to 60mg/24h | 30mg/24h. of diamorphine in a syringe driver converts to ~20mg/24h. of oxycodone in a syringe driver.* |
| Oral oxycodone | s/cut oxycodone | ÷ by 2 or 1.5 | 30mg/24h. of oral oxycodone = 15mg s/cut oxycodone/24h. in a syringe driver. |
| Oral hydromorphone | s/cut hydro-morphone | ÷ by 2 | 16mg/24h. of oral hydromor-phone = 8mg s/cut hydromor-phone/24h. in a syringe driver. |

* It is safer to use the lowest dose and ensure breakthrough medication is available.

## Table 2.5 Opioid dose conversion guide
### Approximate equivalent opioid dose
⚠ Always review the patient regularly after any opioid switch as conversion ratios are approximate

| Oral morphine 24h. total dose (mg) | Oral morphine 4h. dose (mg) | Subcutaneous diamorphine 24h. total dose (mg) | Subcutaneous diamorphine 4h. dose (mg) | Oral oxycodone 24h. total dose (mg) | Oral oxycodone 4h. dose (mg) | Subcutaneous oxycodone 24h. total dose (mg) | Subcutaneous oxycodone 4h. dose (mg) | Oral hydromorphone 24h. total dose (mg) | Oral hydromorphone 4h. dose (mg) | Subcutaneous hydromorphone 24h. total dose (mg) | Subcutaneous alfentanil 24h. total dose (mg) | Subcutaneous morphine 24h. total dose (mg) |
|---|---|---|---|---|---|---|---|---|---|---|---|---|
| 30 | 5 | 10 | 2.5 | 15 | 2.5 | 7.5–10 | 1.25–2.5 | 4 | 1.3 | 2 | 1 | 15 |
| 60 | 10 | 20 | 2.5–5 | 30 | 5 | 15–20 | 2.5–5 | 8 | 1.3 | 4 | 2 | 30 |
| 120 | 20 | 40 | 5–7.5 | 60 | 10 | 30–40 | 5–7.5 | 16 | 2.6 | 8 | 4 | 60 |
| 180 | 30 | 60 | 10 | 90 | 15 | 45–60 | 7.5–10 | 24 | 3.9 | 12 | 6 | 90 |
| 240 | 40 | 80 | 10–15 | 120 | 20 | 60–80 | 10–15 | 32 | 5.2 | 16 | 8 | 120 |
| 360 | 60 | 120 | 20 | 180 | 30 | 90–120 | 15–20 | 48 | 7.8 | 24 | 12 | 180 |

🔵 4-hourly dose may also be used as medication dose for breakthrough pain.

- Conversion doses are approximate only and given as examples
- When changing from one opioid to another, because of toxicity, dose ↳ may be necessary. Review regularly after any changes.
- Be careful with the elderly and patients with renal or significant hepatic impairment – consider reduced doses.
- Breakthrough doses for each opioid are calculated as 1/6 daily dose (i.e. 4-hourly dose) but lower doses may be used if effective.
- Be careful converting opioids at higher doses – lower doses may be necessary due to incomplete cross-tolerance.
- For further advice contact the local palliative care team.

**Table 2.6 Conversion of oral morphine to buprenorphine (Transtec®) patch[1]**

| 24h. oral morphine dose (mg) | Buprenorphine matrix patch (mcgm/h.) replaced every 72h. |
|---|---|
| 30–60 | 35 |
| 61–90 | 52.5 |
| 91–120 | 70 |
| 121–240 | 140 (2×70 patch) |

[1] Source: Summary of product characteristics.

**Table 2.7 Conversion of oral morphine to fentanyl patch**

| 24h. oral morphine dose (mg) | Fentanyl patch strength (mcgm/h.) | 4-hourly oral morphine dose (breakthrough dose) in mg |
|---|---|---|
| 45–134 | 25 | <20 |
| 135–224 | 50 | 25–35 |
| 225–314 | 75 | 40–50 |
| 315–404 | 100 | 55–65 |
| 405–494 | 125 | 70–80 |
| 495–584 | 150 | 85–95 |
| 585–674 | 175 | 100–110 |
| 675–764 | 200 | 115–125 |
| 765–854 | 225 | 130–140 |
| 855–944 | 250 | 145–155 |
| 945–1034 | 275 | 160–170 |
| 1035–1124 | 300 | 175–185 |

**Online converter for fentanyl patches**
🖳 www.globalrph.com/fentconv.htm

**Further information:**
**DTB** Opioid analgesics for cancer pain in primary care. (2005)
**British Pain Society** Recommendations for the appropriate use of opioids in persistent non-cancer pain (2005).
🖳 www.britishpainsociety.org

**Fentanyl:** Selective synthetic opioid.

- Acts on fewer receptors than morphine and so may cause less side effects in some individuals (particularly sedation, cognitive impairment, constipation, myoclonus, and pruritus)
- As it has inactive metabolites and is metabolized mainly in the liver, it is unlikely to cause adverse effects in renal failure
- NEVER attempt dose titration for unstable pain using a fentanyl patch – convert from oral morphine once a stable dose is attained.

**Preparations available:** 📖 p.23

**Conversion from oral morphine to fentanyl patch:** 📖 p.33

**Transdermal Fentanyl patches:** Plasma concentrations peak after 12–24h. so breakthrough doses of opioid are necessary in the first 24h. A depot remains in the skin for ~24h. after the patch is removed.

> ⚠ *Important points*
> - 1:10 patients taking morphine may experience a withdrawal reaction when converted to Fentanyl – give oral morphine on a prn basis to manage withdrawal symptoms for a day or two.
> - Monitor patients using patches if they develop fever or the application site is exposed to external heat. ↑ absorption → ↑ side-effects
> - Fentanyl toxicity is clinically more subtle than morphine toxicity and may present as vagueness, drowsiness, or 'not feeling well'.
> - Sweating ↓ drug absorption by preventing patches sticking to the skin.

**Oral transmucosal Fentanyl lozenges (OTFC):**
- Used for breakthrough pain for patients already on regular strong opioid therapy for chronic pain. Pain relief starts in <10min. and peaks in 20–40min. Lasts 1–3h.
- Start at 200mcgm whatever the background opioid dose. Continue this dose for a further 2 to 3 episodes of breakthrough pain, allowing a 2$^{nd}$ lozenge when necessary to control pain
- If pain is still not controlled,↑ to the next higher dose lozenge
- Continue to titrate in this manner until a dose is found that provides adequate analgesia with minimum adverse effects. New buccal and sublingual preparations of fentanyl are now available

**Buprenorphine:** Opioid agonist and antagonist. It has abuse potential and may cause dependence. It has a much longer duration of action than morphine and sublingually is an effective analgesic for 6–8h. Vomiting may be a problem. Unlike most opioid analgesics, the effects of buprenorphine are only partially reversed by naloxone.

**Preparations available:** 📖 p.23

**Buprenorphine patches:** Buprenorphine patches straddle the weak: strong opioid interface. The maximum dose is 140mcgm/h. (2 × '70') patches) can be used concurrently. Opioids other than buprenorphine can be used for breakthrough pain. NEVER attempt dose titration for unstable pain using a buprenorphine patch – convert from oral morphine once a stable dose is attained (📖 p.31).

## GP Notes:

### Converting from oral morphine to fentanyl patch:[1]

- Give the routine morning dose of modified-release morphine and at the same time apply the appropriate fentanyl patch (📖 p.31)
- No more modified-release morphine should be taken
- Make sure that an appropriate breakthrough dose of immediate-release morphine is available
- Advise patients and relatives that it may take a few days for the fentanyl patch delivery system to stabilize but if there is any increase in pain, there is medicine available to reduce it quickly.

*Example:* If converting from MST® 60mg bd to a fentanyl 25mcgm/h. patch, give the last morning dose of MST® as usual and at the same time apply the fentanyl '25' patch. Make sure that immediate-release morphine 20mg is written up for breakthrough pain to be given 4-hourly as needed (i.e. 1/6 of total 24h morphine dose).

### Converting from a fentanyl patch to modified-release oral morphine:

- Remove the patch early in the day so the patient can be monitored
- Commence the modified-release morphine preparation at the same time
- Calculate the dose using the dose conversion chart (📖 p.30)
- Advise the patient and relatives that while the fentanyl dose reduces and the morphine dose increases, there may be a period of increased drowsiness which should resolve after 24–48h.

*Example:* If converting from fentanyl '75' patch, remove the patch and at the same time commence oral morphine 300mg/24h. in a modified-release preparation.

### Converting from syringe driver diamorphine/morphine to fentanyl patch: Maintain the syringe driver at half strength for 12h. after applying the first patch.

*Example:* Converting from diamorphine 100mg/24h. in a syringe driver – apply a fentanyl '100' patch and restart the syringe driver containing diamorphine 50mg/24h. Stop the syringe driver after 12h. Make sure that breakthrough doses of analgesia are available i.e. diamorphine 15mg s/cut stat (100mg ÷ 6 ≈ 15mg).

### Converting from a fentanyl patch to s/cut diamorphine

Patches create a reservoir of fentanyl in the skin. Blood levels of fentanyl persist for up to 24h. after the patch is removed.

*Example:* After removing a fentanyl '100' patch, replace with diamorphine 60mg/24h. in a syringe driver for the first 24h., then diamorphine 120mg thereafter. Make sure that breakthrough doses of analgesia are available i.e. diamorphine 20mg s/cut stat (120mg ÷ 6 = 20mg).

33

1 Twycross et al. (2002). *Palliative Care Formulary 2.* 2nd edition. Oxford: Radcliffe Medical Press ISBN: 1857755111

# Opioid side effects

**Common side effects of opioid drugs:** Warn all patients about common side effects:

- *Nausea and vomiting* – particularly when first starting medication. Usually wears off within a week. Antiemetics may be needed for 5–7d. e.g. haloperidol 1.5mg nocte. If continues, consider switching to an alternative opioid
- *Constipation* – prescribe prophylactic laxatives e.g. bisacodyl 1–2 tablets nocte. (Fentanyl causes less constipation than morphine)
- *Drowsiness/cognitive impairment* – warn about the dangers of driving, performing other skilled tasks and working with dangerous machinery if affected when starting an opioid or increasing the dose. Usually abates over a few days. Unless severe, continue opioid and wait for drowsiness to wear off. If not improving, consider using an alternative opioid or refer for specialist advice.

## Other less common side effects:

- Difficulty with micturition
- Ureteric spasm
- Biliary spasm
- Dry mouth
- Sweating
- Pruritus
- Headache
- Facial flushing
- Vertigo
- Brady- or tachycardia ± palpitations
- Postural hypotension
- Hypothermia
- Hallucinations
- Mood changes
- Dependence
- Pupillary constriction
- Decreased libido or impotence
- Rashes, urticaria, and pruritus

! Always ensure opioid doses are carefully titrated ('fine-tuned') to maximize analgesia and minimize side effects.

## General management

A number of different approaches may be used to manage persistent opioid-related side effects:

- Treat the side effect e.g. with 5-HT$_3$ antagonists (such as ondansetron) for itching
- Use an alternative opioid
- Use an alternative analgesic method

⚠ If unacceptable toxicity occurs, ↓ the dose. The patient may need to miss several doses and restart at a lower dose.

**Opioid toxicity:** Intentional or unintentional overdose produces:
- Drowsiness or coma
- Confusion – including auditory and/or visual hallucinations
- Vomiting
- Respiratory depression
  - *If respiratory rate ≥8/min. and the patient is easily rousable and not cyanosed* – adopt a policy of 'wait and see'; consider reducing or omitting the next regular dose of opioid. Stop syringe drivers temporarily to allow plasma levels to ↓, then restart at a lower dose
  - *If respiratory rate < 8/min., and the patient is barely rousable/unconscious and/or cyanosed* – dilute a standard ampoule containing naloxone 400mcgm to 10ml with sodium chloride 0.9%. Administer 2ml (80mcg) IV every 2min. until respiratory status is satisfactory to a maximum of 10mg naloxone. If respiratory function still does not improve, question diagnosis. Further boluses may be necessary once respiratory function improves as naloxone is shorter acting than morphine.
- Pinpoint pupils
- Hypotension
- Muscle rigidity/myoclonus – consider renal failure (can produce myoclonus alone). Treat by rehydration, stopping other medication which may exacerbate myoclonus, switching opioid or with clonazepam 2–4mg/24h. depending on circumstances.

**Opioid toxicity may be increased by**
- Dehydration
- Renal failure
- Other change in disease status e.g. hepatic function, weight loss
- Other analgesics e.g. NSAIDs
- Co-administration of amitriptyline

35

**Increase in generalized pain:** Hyperalgesia and allodynia have been reported with high-dose opioids. They are usually associated with myoclonus, and any further ↑ in opioid dose may worsen the pain. Substitution of an alternative opioid often resolves the symptoms. Alternatively, reducing the dose and adding a co-analgesic may be useful.

# Other routes of opioid administration

**Topical opioids:** have been mixed with both metronidazole and hydrocolloid gels for treatment of the pain of skin wounds.

**If oral administration is impossible:** Consider:
- Rectal preparations (e.g. morphine suppository)
- Patches (e.g. fentanyl patch)
- Syringe driver (e.g. containing diamorphine)

**Syringe drivers:** Syringe drivers (Figure 2.3) are used to aid drug delivery when the oral route is no longer feasible. Indications include:
- Intractable vomiting
- Severe dysphagia
- Patient too weak to swallow
- Decreased conscious level
- Poor gut absorption (rare)
- Poor patient compliance

### Types of syringe driver

**MS26 Green driver** – dispenses a set number of mm of fluid in a syringe per 24h. i.e. **daily** rate

$$\text{Rate} = \frac{\text{measured 'length of volume' in mm}}{\text{delivery time in days}}$$

e.g. 48mm = 48mm in one day; rate on dial is '48'

**MS16A Blue driver** – dispenses a set number of mm of fluid in a syringe driver per hour. i.e. **hourly** rate

$$\text{Rate} = \frac{\text{measured 'length of volume' in mm}}{\text{delivery time in hours}}$$

e.g. 48mm/24h. = 2mm/h.; rate on dial is '02'

🛑 Each health care trust should use only one type of syringe driver to decrease the risk of dose errors. A newer digital type of syringe driver is being adopted in several trusts across the UK, though the Graseby is still the most common.

### General principles:
- Draw up the prescribed 24h. medication mixed with water for injection as a diluent (unless contraindicated – see below)
- Set the rate on the syringe driver. Rate of delivery is based on a length of fluid in mm per unit time (see above and Figure 2.3 opposite)
- Ensure the diluent used is compatible with the drugs in the syringe driver. The diluent of choice in most cases is water for injection. 0.9% sodium chloride should be used if using:
  - Levomepromazine
  - Diclofenac
  - Octreotide
  - Ondansetron
- Take care when mixing drugs in a syringe driver. Ensure drugs are compatible (📖 pp.194–7). If combining 2 or 3 drugs in a syringe driver, a larger volume of diluent may be needed (e.g. 20 or 30ml syringe). If >3 drugs are needed in a 1 syringe driver, re-assess treatment aims.

⚠ Local policies may differ. Hands-on training is essential. See 🖥 www.pallcare.info.

### Table 2.8 Drugs commonly used in syringe drivers

| Indication | Drugs |
|---|---|
| Nausea and vomiting | Haloperidol 2.5–10mg/24h. |
| | Levomepromazine 5–200mg/24h. (causes sedation in 50% of patients) |
| | Cyclizine 150mg/24h. (may precipitate if mixed with other drugs) |
| | Metoclopramide 30–100mg/24h. |
| | Octeotide 300–600mcgm/24h. (consultant supervision) |
| | Hyoscine butylbromide 20–60mg/24h. |
| Respiratory secretions | Hyoscine hydrobromide 0.6–2.4mg/24h. |
| | Glycopyrronium 0.6–1.2mg/24h. |
| Restlessness and confusion | Haloperidol 5–15mg/24h. |
| | Levomepromazine 50–200mg/24h. |
| | Midazolam 20–100mg/24h. (and fitting) |
| Pain control | Diamorphine – $^1/_3$ dose oral morphine/24h. |
| | Morphine – $^1/_2$ dose oral morphine/24h. |
| | Oxycodone – $^1/_2$ dose oral oxycodone/24h. |

🛈 Subcutaneous infusion solution should be monitored regularly both to check for precipitation (and discolouration) and to ensure the infusion is running at the correct rate.

⚠ Incorrect use of syringe drivers is a common cause of drug errors.

37

### Figure 2.3 Syringe driver

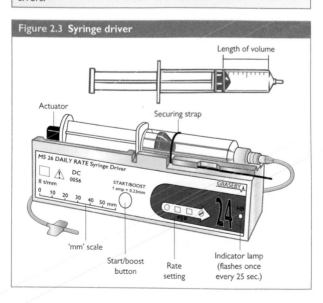

Figure 2.3 Syringe driver

**Morphine conversion:** Diamorphine can be administered subcutaneously in a smaller volume than morphine and, in countries where diamorphine is available, is the preparation of first choice.

| Preparation: | Oral morphine (24h. dose) | Subcutaneous diamorphine | Subcutaneous morphine |
|---|---|---|---|
| Dose ratio: | 3 | 1 | 2 |

When converting opioids other than morphine, calculate the equivalent dose of oral morphine over 24h. (📖 p.31) and continue as above.

**Mixing drugs in a syringe driver:** Drugs that can be mixed with diamorphine include:
- Cyclizine
- Haloperidol
- Hyoscine butylbromide
- Hyoscine hydrobromide
- Metoclopramide
- Ondansetron
- Levomepromazine
- Midazolam
- Octreotide
- Glycopyrronium

🛈 Maximum of 3 drugs in 1 syringe

### Use a separate syringe driver for:
- Dexamethasone (unless <4mg)
- Phenobarbital
- Diclofenac
- Ketamine
- Ketorolac

### Drugs not suitable for subcutaneous usage: *Include:*
- Diazepam
- Chlorpromazine
- Prochlorperazine

### Notes on using cyclizine in a syringe driver:
- Cyclizine is incompatible with 0.9% normal saline
- If dose of cyclizine is >75mg/24h. *in conjunction with* a dose of diamorphine >160mg/24h., dilute to >14ml in a 20ml syringe to ensure the medications remain compatible in the syringe.

### Notes on using levomepromazine in a syringe driver:
- Levomepromazine can be irritant
- If skin site soreness becomes a problem, dilute levomepromazine with 0.9% saline rather than water for injections.

🛈 If diamorphine is combined with levomepromazine, normal saline can only be used when diamorphine concentration is <40mg/ml – if >40mg/ml, use water for injections and either ↑ the size of syringe used or consider adding dexamethasone 1mg to reduce the skin reaction.

**Syringe driver drugs and dosage charts:** 📖 p.37 and pp.194–7

### Further information:
Dickman *et al.* The Syringe Driver: Continuous Subcutaneous Infusions in Palliative Care (2<sup>nd</sup> Edition 2005). OUP ISBN: 019856693X

## GP Notes: Troubleshooting

| | |
|---|---|
| *Infusion running too fast* | Check the rate setting and recalculate. |
| *Infusion running too slow* | Check the start button, battery, syringe driver, and cannula, and make sure the injection site is not inflamed. |
| *Site reaction* | • Cyclizine and levomepromazine cause site reactions most commonly. If there is no alternative to subcutaneous administration it may be helpful to add dexamethasone 1mg to the mixture<br>• Firmness or swelling is not necessarily a problem but change the needle site if there is pain or obvious inflammation<br>• A plastic/teflon needle may reduce local irritation if the patient has nickle allergy. |
| *Precipitation* | • Check compatibility of drugs<br>• Check solution regularly for precipitation and dis-colouration – discard if it occurs<br>• Cyclizine may precipitate at high doses, particularly in combination with high doses of diamorphine<br>• Other combinations may also cause cloudiness in the syringe<br>• On rare occasions a patient may need 2 or 3 separate syringe drivers to separate the drugs. |
| *Light flashing* | This is normal. The light flashes:<br>• BLUE – once per second<br>• GREEN – once per 25 second<br><br>Flashing stops when the battery needs changing. The syringe driver continues to operate for 24h. after the light has stopped flashing. |
| *Alarm* | Always sounds when the battery is inserted. Silence by pressing the 'Start/Test' button.<br>If alarm sounds at any other time, check for:<br>• Empty syringe<br>• Kinked tube<br>• Blocked needle/tubing<br>• Jammed plunger |

# Neuropathic pain

Neuropathic pain occurs as a result of damage to neural tissue. Examples include post-herpetic neuralgia, complex regional pain syndrome (reflex sympathetic dystrophy), peripheral neuropathy (e.g. due to DM), compression neuropathy, and phantom limb pain.

Pain typically occurs in association with altered sensation e.g. burning, stabbing, or numbness. Pain may also be provoked by non-noxious stimuli (allodynia) e.g. gentle heat or cold.

Neuropathic pain is generally managed with tricyclic antidepressants or antiepileptic drugs.

## Tricyclic antidepressants

**Amitriptyline:** is prescribed most frequently (unlicensed indication). Start at a dose of 25mg nocte – 10mg nocte if elderly. Increase dose by 10–25mg nocte every 5–7d. to a maximum of 75mg nocte as needed (higher doses under specialist supervision).

### Alternatives include:
* Nortriptyline – also given at an initial dose of 10–25mg nocte – may produce fewer side effects than amitriptyline
* Dosulepin – 25–75mg nocte
* Lofepramine – particularly suitable for the elderly/frail – start at 70mg nocte increasing to 70mg bd as necessary after 5–7d.

## Anticonvulsants

**Gabapentin and pregabalin:** Both licensed for treatment of neuropathic pain. Dosage regimens:
* *Gabapentin*: 300mg on day 1; 300mg bd on day 2; 300mg tds on day 3; then increase dose according to response in steps of 300mg daily – in 3 divided doses – to a maximum of 1.8g/d.
* *Pregabalin*: Initially 50mg/d. in 2–3 divided doses, increased if necessary after 3–7d. to 300mg daily in 2–3 divided doses, increased further if necessary after 7d. to a maximum of 600mg daily in 2–3 divided doses. Drowsiness has been reported especially if given in combination with opioids such as oxycodone.

**Carbamazepine:** Unlicensed and often poorly tolerated. Start with 100–200mg 1–2x/d. (less if elderly or frail). Build up dose slowly to minimize adverse effects to the usual dose of 0.8–1.2g daily in divided doses. Oxcarbazine is an alternative for trigeminal neuralgia.

**Sodium valproate, lamotrigine, and phenytoin:** Are also occasionally used for neuropathic pain but are reserved for use under specialist supervision.

**NSAIDs:** Sometimes effective for neuropathic pain – either because there is mixed nociceptive pain or due to ↓ inflammatory sensitization of nerves. There is considerable variation in individual patient tolerance and response (📖 p.20).

**Opioids:** Neuropathic pain often responds only partially to opioid analgesics. Of the opioids, oxycodone, tramadol and methadone are probably the most effective – consider when other measures fail.

## Other drug treatments

**Capsaicin:** is a topical treatment licensed for neuropathic pain. Apply a small amount 3–4x/d. Acts by counter-irritation – but intense burning during initial treatment limits use. Advise patients to wash hands after application and avoid application after a hot shower/bath (↑ burning sensation).

**Corticosteroids:** may help relieve pressure in compression neuropathy and, indirectly, pain. Start with a high initial dose to achieve rapid results (dexamethasone 8mg/d. works in 1–3d.), then rapidly ↓ dose to the minimum that maintains benefit.

**Ketamine or lidocaine:** by intravenous infusion (both unlicensed) have been used in specialist centres for some forms of neuropathic pain.

Lidocaine patches 5% are licensed for use in post-herpetic neuralgia. They should be applied in the affected area on unbroken skin, and it is recommended that they not be used for more than 12 hours in 24. These patches have been used for a variety of unlicensed neuropathic pain scenarios in the palliative care setting.

## Non-drug treatments:

- Patients with chronic neuropathic pain often require a multidisciplinary approach including physiotherapy and psychological support
- TENS and/or acupuncture help in some cases (🕮 p.202)
- Nerve blocks, and/or central electrical stimulation may help in some cases – refer for specialist advice.

**Referral:** If unable to achieve adequate pain relief, consider referral to a specialist pain control clinic (or palliative care team if more appropriate).

**Trigeminal neuralgia:** 🕮 p.60

**Post-herpetic neuralgia:** 🕮 p.60

**Diabetic neuropathy:** 🕮 p.61

## Further information:

British Pain Society Recommendations for the appropriate use of opioids in persistent non-cancer pain (2005).
🖥 www.britishpainsociety.org

---

**Advice for patients: Further information**

Neuropathy Trust 🖥 www.neurocentre.com

# Spiritual pain

*"The realization that life is likely to end soon may well give rise to feelings of the unfairness of what is happening, and at much of what has gone before, and, above all, a desolate feeling of meaninglessness. Here lies, I believe, the essence of spiritual pain."*

Dame Cicely Saunders (1918–2005)

**Spirituality:** Central to the problematic nature of 'spiritual care' is how 'spirituality' is defined.

- A definition that *includes* religious elements may cause a sense of exclusion among those who hold to a different belief system
- A definition that *excludes* all religious elements may exclude those within society who subscribe to a particular belief

A more functional definition is that spirituality is what we do with our pain, e.g. how we respond when life does not go as we plan.

**Spiritual needs:** It may be suggested that the spirit manifests itself through the expression of its needs:

- To find meaning, purpose in life, suffering, and death
- For hope and creativity
- A belief and love in self, others and a power beyond the self
- To find forgiveness and acceptance
- To be listened to with respect
- For a source of hope and strength
- For trust
- For expression of personal beliefs and values
- For spiritual practices

**Spiritual pain:** Manifested by a deep sense of hurt stemming from feelings of loss or separation from one's God or deity, a sense of personal inadequacy, and/or a lasting condition of loneliness of spirit. Components include:

- Lack of meaning (why me?)
- Hopelessness or despair
- Feelings of emptiness
- Feelings of injustice
- Pointlessness
- Powerlessness
- Feelings of being abandoned
- Spiritual guilt
- Anxiety/fear of God (What will happen after death?)

**Spiritual care:** Relevant to all aspects of a patient's care. Essential skills include:

- Empathic and active listening
- Good communication
- Helping patients to deal with past, present, and future issues
- Not feeling obliged to do something to provide care

## GP Notes:

**Principles of spiritual care:** Having no solution is not the same as having no response:

| Action | Reaction |
|--------|----------|
| *Foster realistic hope:* To give unrealistic hope that life will be prolonged is unethical, but there is always something more that can be done to bolster hope in a realistic way. | *Presence:* To be maximally useful to patients and their experiences, we must be aware of our own biases and distortions. |
| *Create 'space' for patients:* Patients need to feel they still have some choice and control. | *Listen attentively* with genuineness and acceptance. |
| *Combine professionalism with compassion* | *Facilitate exploration:* Meaning cannot be given by another, it must be found by the person him/herself. |
| *Remain in touch with your own spiritual needs* | *Allow for mystery:* Some issues will always defy explanation. |
| | *Allow for paradox:* Conflicting priorities in the care of patients may mean that some questions are difficult to answer. The emotional pain of this needs to be recognized and supported. |

### Advice for patients: Experience of diagnosis of lung cancer

43

'When I was diagnosed with lung cancer, in the space of a few days everything changed. I had to stop working. I began chemotherapy, which made me tired. At home, instead of being the person who provided for my wife and children, they were having to look after me. I felt myself to be nothing more than a burden, no longer fit to be a husband, or father. I just felt that I might as well be dead.'

# Prescribing for patients with renal impairment

It is common for patients with chronic pain to have co-existent renal failure. Renal function ↓ with age but may not be reflected by raised creatinine due to ↓ muscle mass. Always assume mild to moderate renal failure if prescribing for the elderly.

**Degree of renal impairment:** Estimated glomerular filtration rate (eGFR), based on serum creatinine, age, gender and ethnic origin, is now provided to GPs when renal function tests are done.

- *Mild renal impairment* – eGFR 60–89ml/min/1.73m$^2$
- *Moderate renal impairment* – eGFR 30–59ml/min/1.73m$^2$
- *Severe renal impairment* – eGFR <30ml/min/1.73m$^2$

**Results of renal impairment:** Drug effects are altered by:

- *Inability to excrete the drug* – may cause toxicity. Dose reduction or increase in the interval between doses may be necessary
- *Increased sensitivity to drugs* – even if elimination is unimpaired
- *Poor tolerance of side effects* – nephrotoxic drugs may have more serious side effects
- *Reduced effectiveness*

**Pain relieving drugs:**

- *Paracetamol:* Is safe in renal failure but reduce dose to 3g/d. if the patient has severe renal impairment. Paracetamol is removed by haemodialysis but not by peritoneal dialysis
- *NSAIDs:* Avoid if possible in patients with renal impairment. Where use is essential, sulindac is the NSAID of choice as it has renal-sparing effects. These effects are lost with doses >100mg bd. In patients on dialysis, NSAIDs may be used if kidney protection is no longer an issue
- *Codeine and dihydrocodeine:* There is an increase in CNS side effects in renal failure – particularly drowsiness. Use with care either in combined preparations (e.g. co-codamol) or alone.
- *Morphine, diamorphine, and hydromorphone:* Metabolites of morphine/hydromorphone accumulate in renal failure and cause ↑ incidence of neurotoxic side effects e.g. myoclonus and confusion. Avoid long-acting preparations
- *Oxycodone:* 90% metabolized by the liver. For patients with mild or moderate renal failure, oxycodone can be used with caution, so long as the dose is titrated up slowly. Contraindicated in severe renal impairment because the 10% normally excreted unchanged in the urine, may then accumulate
- *Fentanyl and alfentanil:* Mainly metabolized in the liver to inactive metabolites. Short half-life. Licensed for use in renal failure. Specialist advice is recommended when changing patients from subcutaneous diamorphine to subcutaneous alfentanil.

**Haemodialysis:** May produce significant falls in morphine concentration leading to pain during or shortly after dialysis.

**Further information:**

BNF – Appendix 3
Patients on dialysis – consult local renal unit.

**Table 2.9** Dosage of commonly used pain-relieving drugs for patients with renal impairment

| | Renal failure | | |
|---|---|---|---|
| Drug | Mild | Moderate | Severe |
| Paracetamol | Normal dose | Normal dose | ↓ dose to 1g tds |
| NSAIDs | Normal dose | Avoid if possible | Avoid unless on haemodialysis |
| **Weak opioids** | | | |
| Co-codamol/ co-dydramol | Normal dose | 6 tablets/24h. | 4 tablets/24h. |
| Codeine/ dihydrocodeine | Normal dose | 15–30mg tds | 15mg tds or qds |
| Tramadol | Normal dose | 50–100mg bd | 50mg bd |
| **Strong opioids** | | | |
| Morphine | 75% normal dose | 2.5–5mg 4-hourly | 1.25–2.5mg 4-hourly |
| Diamorphine | Normal dose | Normal dose | 2.5mg s/cut tds* |
| Hydromorphone | Normal dose | 1.3mg* | 1.3mg* |
| Oxycodone | 2.5mg qds or 5mg bd* | 2.5mg qds or 5mg bd* | Avoid |
| Fentanyl | Normal dose | 75% normal dose* | 50% normal dose* |
| **Other drugs** | | | |
| Amitriptyline | Normal dose | Normal dose | Normal dose |
| Gabapentin | 300mg bd | 300mg od | 300mg alternate days |
| Baclofen | 5mg tds | 5mg bd | 5mg od |

*Titrate dose

# Chapter 3

# Specific non-malignant pain scenarios

# Irritable bowel syndrome (IBS)

Irritable bowel syndrome (IBS) is a chronic (>6mo.) relapsing and remitting condition of unknown cause with symptoms including: Abdominal pain or discomfort; Bloating; and Change in bowel habit.

It is a diagnosis of exclusion with no confirmatory test and no cure. Extremely common. Lifetime prevalence ≥ 20%, though ~ 75% never consult a GP. ♀>♂ (2.5:1). Symptoms can appear at any age.

**Diagnosis of IBS:** Abdominal pain or discomfort that is:
- relieved by defaecation, or
- associated with altered bowel frequency or stool form

*and* ≥2 of the following:
- altered stool passage (straining, urgency, incomplete evacuation)
- abdominal bloating (♀>♂), distension, tension or hardness
- symptoms made worse by eating
- passage of mucus

*Other commonly associated symptoms include:* lethargy, nausea, backache and bladder symptoms.

**Differential diagnosis:**
- Colonic carcinoma
- Coeliac disease
- Inflammatory bowel disease (Crohn's disease or UC)
- Pelvic inflammatory disease
- Endometriosis
- GI infection
- Thyrotoxicosis

**Investigation:** A diagnosis of exclusion. How far to investigate is a clinical judgement weighing risks of investigation against possibility of serious disease. Judgement is based on age of the patient, family history, length of history and symptom cluster.
- *Patients <40y.:* Check FBC, ESR, and antibody testing to exclude coeliac disease
- *Patients >40y.:* Colonic cancer must be excluded for any patient with a persistent, unexplained change in bowel habit - particularly towards looser stools.
- *Other investigations to consider:*
  - Thyroid function tests if other symptoms/signs of thyroid disease
  - Stool samples to exclude GI infection if diarrhoea
  - Endocervical swabs for *Chlamydia*
  - Colonoscopy to exclude inflammatory bowel disease
  - Laparoscopy to exclude endometriosis

**Referral:** to gastroenterology/general surgery if:
- Passing blood (except if from an anal fissure or haemorrhoids) – U
- Abdominal, rectal or pelvic mass – U
- Unintentional/unexplained weight loss – U/S
- Positive inflammatory markers and/or anaemia- U/S
- >40y. with new symptoms – U (if age >60y.)/S/R
- Change in symptoms – especially if >40y. – U (if age >60y.)/S/R
- Atypical features (i.e. not those listed above) – U/S/R
- Family history of bowel or ovarian cancer – R
- Patient is unhappy to accept a diagnosis of IBS despite explanation – R

U=urgent; S=soon; R=routine.

**Treatment:** Reassure. Information leaflets are helpful. Encourage effective use of leisure time and regular physical exercise.

**Diet:** Encourage patients to have regular meals and take time to eat. Avoid missing meals or leaving long gaps between eating
● Drink ≥8 cups of fluid/d., especially water. Restrict tea/coffee to 3 cups/d. ↓ intake of alcohol and fizzy drinks.
● ↓ intake of high-fibre food (e.g.wholemeal/high-fibre flour and breads, cereals high in bran, and whole grains such as brown rice).
● ↓ intake of 'resistant starch' found in processed or re-cooked foods.
● Limit fresh fruit to 3×80g portions/d.
● For diarrhoea, avoid sorbitol, an artificial sweetener.
● For wind and bloating consider increasing intake of oats (e.g. oat-based breakfast cereal or porridge) and linseeds (≤ 1 tablespoon/d.).
● Up to 50% may be helped by exclusion of certain foods (especially patients with diarrhoea - predominant disease). Diaries may help identify foods that provoke symptoms. Common candidates are dairy products, citrus fruits, caffeine, alcohol, tomatoes, gluten, and eggs. Refer to dietician for exclusion diet.

**Specific measures:**
● *Probiotics:* Some evidence of effectiveness. Try a 4 wk. trial of treatment.
● *Fibre / bulking agents:* Constipation-predominant IBS. Bran can make some patients worse. Ispaghula husk is better tolerated. Laxatives are an alternative but avoid use of lactulose.
● *Antispasmodics:* e.g. mebeverine, peppermint oil. All equally effective. If no response in a few days, switch to another - different agents suit different individuals. Once symptoms are controlled use prn dosing.
● *Antidiarrhoeal preparations:* e.g. loperamide. Avoid codeine phosphate as may cause dependence. Use prn for patients with diarrhoea - predominant disease. Use pre-emptive doses to cover difficult situations (e.g. air travel).
● *Antidepressants:* There is evidence that low dose amitriptyline e.g. 10mg nocte is effective. SSRIs are less effective unless the patient is overtly depressed. Withdraw if no response after 4-6wk.
● *Psychotherapy and hypnosis:* Some effect in trials. Reserve for cases that have failed to respond to more conventional treatment.

**Failure to respond to treatment:** Consider another diagnosis - review history and examination ± refer for further investigation.

**Prognosis:** >50% still have symptoms after 5y.

**Further information:**
NICE Irritable bowel syndrome in adults: diagnosis and management of irritable bowel syndrome in primary care (2008) 🖳 www.nice.org.uk

**Advice and support for patients:**
**The Gut Trust** ☎ 0114 272 32 53 🖳 www.theguttrust.org

49

# Pelvic pain

**History:** Timing and quality of pain, precipitating and relieving factors, relationship to menstrual cycle (and possibility of pregnancy), dyspareunia, bowel and bladder symptoms, history of ectopic pregnancy, pelvic infection or surgery, psychological problems.

**Examination:** Abdominal (including rectal examination), pelvic and vaginal examination (with smear if overdue). Normal pelvic and vaginal examination makes a gynaecological cause unlikely.

**Management:**

*Acute pelvic pain:* Admit unless cause is known and ectopic pregnancy can be excluded.

*Chronic pelvic pain:* On the basis of history and examination decide whether or not the cause is gynaecological – patients with gynaecological causes usually have dyspareunia and the pain may be cyclical.
- If gynaecological, arrange pelvic USS. Most patients will also need laparoscopy – refer
- If GI pain, consider colonoscopy or barium studies
- Other investigations: urine – MSU (and dipstick for red cells); IVP; spine X-ray.

## Chronic pelvic pain

**Mittelschmerz:** Midcycle pain that occurs around the time of ovulation. Reassure.

**Endometriosis:**[G] Presence of tissue histologically similar to endometrium outside the uterine cavity and myometrium. Most commonly found in the pelvis but can occur anywhere. Affects ~1:5 women.
- *Risk factors:* age, family history, heavy periods, frequent cycles. Oral contraceptives and pregnancy are protective
- *History:* Pelvic pain (cyclical ± non-cyclical), dyspareunia, dysmenorrhoea, infertility, menorrhagia
- *Examination:* Pelvic tenderness, pelvic mass, fixation of uterus, tender nodules can occasionally be felt on the utero-sacral ligaments
- *Investigation:* refer to gynaecology for laparoscopy/transvaginal USS.

*Management:*
- Infertility – refer for gynaecology/infertility opinion
- Cyclical pain – NSAID prn from first day of period
- Constant pain, dyspareunia or cyclical pain unresponsive to NSAID – progestogen (e.g. norethisterone 10–15mg/d. for 4–6mo.) or continuous COC (4 packets without break then 7d. break – effective in 70–80% of patients)
- If symptoms are not controlled – refer. GnRH agonists e.g. goserelin may be used but side effects can be troublesome. Surgical options include laparoscopy or laparotomy with ablation of lesions and division of adhesions; tubal surgery; hysterectomy.

🛈 For all forms of treatment there is a recurrence rate of 15–20%.
- If relapse in <6mo., consider treatment has failed and try an alternative
- If relapse >6mo. after treatment, consider a relapse and repeat.

**Pelvic venous congestion:** Pelvic veins become dilated and congested. Treatment is with continuous progestogens.

**Pelvic inflammatory disease (PID):** Common causes include chlamydia and gonorrhoea infections. Acute PID may be asymptomatic. >10% of patients develop tubal infertility after 1 episode; 50% after 3 episodes. Risk of ectopic pregnancy ↑ x10 after a single episode. Chronic PID, causing chronic pelvic pain results from inadequately treated acute PID.

- *History:* Pain and dyspareunia, menorrhagia, dysmenorrhoea.
- *Examination:* Generalized lower abdominal/pelvic tenderness, cervical excitation, adnexal mass.
- *Investigation:* Screen for chlamydial and gonorrhoeal infection. A negative result does not exclude diagnosis.
- *Management:* Treat acute PID with antibiotics in accordance with current BNF recommendation. If chronic PID is suspected, or chronic pelvic pain with no obvious cause, refer to gynaecology. Once diagnosis is confirmed, treatment options include long-term antibiotics or surgery.

**Psychological causes of pelvic pain:** These do occur but be careful not to dismiss organic symptoms as psychological. Psychological pain may be a consequence of, and perpetuate, physical pain. Diagnosis is one of exclusion.

**Psychological support:** Many women will have had pain for years. Often there is delay in diagnosis of the cause – and, frequently, they have been told that their pain is psychosomatic. Be sympathetic and supportive and use a co-operative strategy for management.

### Table 3.1 Causes of pelvic pain

| Gynaecological | | Non-gynaecological | |
|---|---|---|---|
| **Acute** | **Chronic** | **Acute** | **Chronic** |
| Ectopic pregnancy | Endometriosis | Appendicitis | Irritable bowel syndrome |
| Infection | Adhesions | Cystitis | Musculoskeletal |
| Endometriosis | Fibroids | Neurological | Psychological |
| Torsion of fibroid | Ovarian cyst | Colitis | Bowel or bladder cancer |
| Dysmenorrhoea | Venous congestion | Psychological | Neurological |
| Ovarian cyst (torsion, bleeding or rupture) | PID | | |

### Further information:

**Royal College of Obstetricians and Gynaecology (RCOG)**
🖳 www.rcog.org.uk
- Chronic pelvic pain: initial management (2006)
- The investigation and management of endometriosis (2006)

### Advice for patients: Information and support

🖳 www.hysterectomy-association.org.uk/
🖳 www.womenshealthlondon.org.uk/
**Pelvic Pain Support Network** 🖳 www.pelvicpain.org.uk
**National Endometriosis Society** ☎ 0808 808 2227
🖳 www.endo.org.uk

# Headache and facial pain

Common presenting complaint in general practice. The skill lies in deciding which headaches are benign needing no intervention, and which require action.

## History:

- *Does the patient have >1 type of headache?* If so, take a separate history for each
- *Time:* When did the headaches start? New or recently changed headache calls for especially careful assessment. How often do they happen? Do they have any pattern? (e.g. constant, episodic, daily) How long do they last? Why is the patient coming to the doctor now?
- *Character:* Nature and quality, site and spread of the pain. Associated symptoms e.g. nausea/vomiting, visual disturbance, photophobia, neurological symptoms
- *Cause:* Predisposing and/or trigger factors; aggravating and/or relieving factors; family history
- *Response:* Details of medication used (type, dose, frequency, timing). What does the patient do? e.g. can the patient continue work?
- *Health between attacks:* Do the headaches go completely or does the patient still feel unwell between attacks?
- *Anxieties and concerns* of the patient.

**Examination:** *In acute, severe headache, examine for purpuric skin rash. In all cases check BP, brief neurological examination including fundi, visual acuity and gait, palpation of the temporal region/sinuses for tenderness, and examination of the neck. In young children measure head circumference and plot on a centile chart*

### ⚠ Red flags:

- New/unexpected headache
- Thunderclap headache
- Aura for first time and using COC
- New onset age >50y. or <10y.
- New onset in a patient with a history of HIV or cancer
- Headache with atypical aura (>1h. ± motor weakness)
- Progressive headache, worsening over weeks
- Associated postural change

**Investigation:** Often not needed. Consider ESR if temporal arteritis is suspected.

**Management:** Direct treatment at cause.

**Differential diagnosis:** Table 3.2. ⓘ ↑BP may cause acute or chronic headache.

**Meningism:** Headache, stiff neck and photophobia. Associated with meningitis. May also be seen with encephalitis and subarachnoid haemorrhage (SAH).

**Facial pain:** Treat the cause. *Common causes include:* trigeminal neuralgia; temporomandibular joint disorders; dental disorders; sinusitis; migrainous neuralgia; shingles and post-herpetic neuralgia.

No cause is found in many patients – it is then termed *atypical facial pain.* Atypical facial pain may respond to simple analgesia with paracetamol or a NSAID. If this fails, try nerve painkillers e.g. amitriptyline nocte. Refer those with troublesome symptoms to ENT, maxillofacial surgery, or neurology.

## Table 3.2 Differential diagnosis of headache

|  | Cause | Features | Management |
|---|---|---|---|
| Acute new headache | Meningitis | Fever, photophobia, stiff neck, rash, photophobia | IV or IM phenoxy-methylpenicillin and immediate admission |
|  | Encephalitis | Fever, confusion, ↓ conscious level | Immediate admission |
|  | Subarachnoid haemorrhage | 'Thunder-clap' or very sudden onset headache ± stiff neck | Immediate admission |
|  | Head injury | Bruising/injury; ↓ conscious level, periods of lucidity, amnesia | Consider admission |
|  | Sinusitis | Tender over sinuses ± history of upper respiratory tract infection (URTI) | Steam inhalation, antibiotics and/or steroid nasal spray |
|  | Dental caries | Facial pain ± tenderness | Consider antibiotics. Refer to dentist |
|  | Tropical illness | History of travel, fever | Consider admission |
| Acute recurrent headache | Migraine | Aura, visual disturbance, nausea/vomiting, triggers | 📖 p.56 |
|  | Cluster headache | Nightly pain in one eye for 2–3mo. then pain free for >1y. | 📖 p.59 |
|  | Exertional or coital headache | Suggested by history of association | NSAID or propranolol before attacks |
|  | Trigeminal neuralgia | Intense stabbing pain lasting seconds in trigeminal nerve distribution | 📖 p.61 |
|  | Glaucoma | Red eye, haloes, ↓ visual acuity, pupil abnormality | Refer to ophthalmology |
| Subacute headache | Temporal (giant cell) arteritis | >50y., scalp tenderness, ↑ ESR, rarely ↓ visual acuity | 📖 p.59 |
| Chronic headache | Tension-type headache | Band around the head, stress, low mood | 📖 p.58 |
|  | Cervicogenic headache | Unilateral or bilateral; band from neck to forehead; scalp tenderness | Treat with NSAIDs ± paracetamol ± physiotherapy |
|  | Medication overuse headache | Rebound headache on stopping analgesics | 📖 p.58 |
|  | ↑ intracranial pressure | Worse on waking/sneezing, neurological signs, ↑BP, ↓ pulse rate | Same day neurology referral |
|  | Paget's disease | >40y., bowed tibia, ↑ alk phos | Refer to rheumatology |

# Migraine

Migraine affects 10% of the UK population. ♂:♀≈1:2. It is more than just a headache. Attacks can force the patient to abandon everyday activities for several days. Even in symptom-free periods, patients may live in fear of the next attack. 1:3 sufferers will experience significant disability as a result of their migraines at some stage of their lives.

**Cause:** Disturbance of cerebral blood flow under the influence of 5-HT.

**Clinical picture:** Three common types:
- *Aura* – aura alone with no headache – visual chaos (e.g. zig-zag lines, jumbling of print, dots); hemianopia; hemiparesis; dysphasia; dyspraxia; dysarthria; ataxia (basilar migraine)
- *Classical migraine* – aura lasting 10–30min. followed by unilateral throbbing headache ± nausea or vomiting ± photophobia
- *Episodic migraine (common migraine)* – unilateral throbbing headache ± nausea or vomiting ± photophobia but without aura – often premenstrual.

**Criteria for diagnosis if no aura:** ≥5 headaches lasting 4–72h. + nausea/vomiting or photophobia/phonophobia and ≥2 of following:

- Unilateral headache
- Pulsating headache
- Moderate/severe pain intensity
- Interferes with normal functioning
- ↑ by climbing stairs/other routine activities

**History, examination, and differential diagnosis:** 📖 pp.52–3

**Trigger factors:** 50% of patients have a trigger for their migraine. Consider:
- *Psychological factors:* Stress/relief of stress; anxiety/depression; extreme emotions e.g. anger or grief
- *Food factors:* Lack of food/infrequent meals; foods containing monosodium glutamate, caffeine and tyramine; specific foods e.g. chocolate, citrus fruits, cheese, alcohol, especially red wine
- *Sleep:* Overtiredness (physical/mental); changes in sleep patterns (e.g. late nights, weekend lie-in, shift work, holidays); long-distance travel
- *Environmental factors:* Loud noise, bright/flickering lights, strong perfume, stuffy atmosphere, VDUs, strong winds, extreme heat/cold
- *Health factors:* Hormonal changes (e.g. monthly periods, COC pill, HRT, the menopause); ↑BP; toothache or pain in the eyes, sinuses or neck; unaccustomed physical activity.

**Assessing severity:** Assessment scales such as the MIDAS scale (opposite) can be useful in assessing impact of symptoms on daily life and monitoring response to treatment.

**Management:** 📖 p.56

The migraine disability assessment score is reproduced with permission of the British Association for the Study of Headache (BASH) Headache Guidelines 2003. 🖳 www.bash.org.uk.

**Migraine disability assessment score (MIDAS):** Used to assess the impact of migraine symptoms on lifestyle.

**Instructions:** Please answer the following questions about ALL the headaches you have had over the last 3mo. If you did not do the activity in the last 3mo. write 0.

| | |
|---|---|
| 1. On how many days in the last 3mo. did you miss work or school because of your headache? | ☐ days |
| 2. How many days in the last 3mo. was your productivity at work or school ↓ by ≥½ because of your headaches? *(Do not include days you counted in question 1 where you missed work or school)* | ☐ days |
| 3. On how many days in the last 3mo. did you not do household work* because of your headache? | ☐ days |
| 4. How many days in the last 3mo. was your productivity in household work ↓ by ≥½ because of your headaches? *(Do not include days you counted in question 3 where you did not do household work)* | ☐ days |
| 5. On how many days in the last 3mo. did you miss family, social, or leisure activities because of your headaches? | ☐ days |
| **MIDAS score TOTAL** | ☐ days |
| A. On how many days in the last 3mo. did you have a headache? *(If a headache lasted more than 1 day, count each day)* | ☐ days |
| B. On a scale of 0–10, on average how painful were these headaches? *(Where 0 = no pain at all, and 10 = pain as bad as can it be)* | ☐ |

Questions A and B measure the frequency of the migraine and the severity of pain. They are not used to reach the MIDAS score, but provide extra information helpful for making treatment decisions.

### Interpreting the MIDAS score

| | | | |
|---|---|---|---|
| I | Score: 0–5 | Minimal/infrequent disability | Tend to have little or no treatment needs. Can often manage with OTC medication. If infrequent severe attacks, may require triptan. |
| II | Score: 6–10 | Mild/infrequent disability | May require medication for acute attacks e.g. NSAID ± antiemetic or triptan. |
| III | Score: 11–20 | Moderate disability | Will need medication for acute attacks. Consider prophylaxis. Consider other causes for headaches e.g. tension type headache. |
| IV | Score: ≥21 | Severe disability | |

* Unpaid work such as housework, shopping and caring for children and others.

**Management:** Aim to control symptoms and minimize their impact on the patient's life.

> **Management of an acute attack[G]:** *Advise to rest* in a quiet, dark place and sleep if possible. Use a treatment ladder. Step up if 3 failures at any one step.
> - *Step 1: Oral analgesic and anti-emetic:* aspirin 600–900mg or ibuprofen 400–600mg ± prochlorperazine 3–6mg bd or domperidone 10mg qds
> - *Step 2: Rectal analgesic ± antiemetic:* diclofenac 100mg (maximum 200mg/24h.) + domperidone 30–60mg (maximum 120mg/24h.)
> - *Step 3: Specific anti-migraine drugs:* e.g. sumatriptan 50–100mg po, 20mg nasal spray, or 6mg s/cut - not effective if taken before the headache develops - stops 70–85% attacks - start with lowest dose and ↑ as needed - do not give if ergotamine taken <24h. previously.
> - *Step 4: Combinations:* e.g. sumatriptan 50mg + naproxen 500mg

### If called to see a patient with an acute attack:
- Administer IM diclofenac 75mg ± IM chlorpromazine 25–50mg
- Alternatively, consider 5-HT$_1$ agonist e.g. sumatriptan unless 2 injections/tablets/nasal sprays already given in last 24h. or ergotamine in <24h.
- Admit if becoming dehydrated.

**Treatment of recurrence within the same attack:** Repeat symptomatic treatments within their dose limitations – pre-emptively if recurrence is usual/expected. If using triptans, a 2$^{nd}$ dose may be effective, but repeated dosing can cause rebound headache. Naratriptan and eletriptan are associated with relatively low recurrence rates.

### Management of chronic migraine:
- Reassure about the benign nature of migraine
- Instruct patients about management of an acute attack
- Ask the patient to keep a diary to identify possible trigger factors, assess headache frequency, severity and response to treatment
- Avoid trigger factors where possible. Give advice on relaxation techniques and stress management to all patients
- Stop the COC pill if migraine starts or worsens when the pill is started – especially if focal symptoms develop
- Consider prophylaxis if frequent or very severe attacks

**Prophylaxis:** Consider if ≥4 attacks/mo. or severe attacks. ↓ attacks by ~50%. Try a drug for 2mo. before deeming it ineffective. If effective, continue for 4–6mo. then ↓ dose slowly before stopping.
- *1$^{st}$ line:* β-blocker e.g. atenolol 25–100mg bd or TCA e.g. amitriptyline 10–150mg 1–2h. before bed – start at low dose and ↑ dose every 2–4wk
- *2$^{nd}$ line:* Topiramate 25–50mg od/bd; sodium valproate 300mg–1g bd.
- *3$^{rd}$ line:* Gabapentin 300mg od – 800mg tds; methysergide 1–2mg tds
- *Others:* limited/uncertain effect – pizotifen, clonidine, verapamil, SSRIs

**Alternative therapies:** Feverfew 200mg daily – some evidence of effectiveness after use for 6wk. Acupuncture may also be helpful.

## GP Notes: Tips for managing menstrual migraine

Consider:
- *NSAIDs* e.g. mefenamic acid 500mg tds/qds from onset of menstruation to last day of bleeding
- *Transdermal oestrogen* e.g. transdermal oestrogen 100mcgm – apply 3d. before period and continue for 7d. (⚠ avoid in focal migraine)
- *Women on COC pill:* Running 3 packets back to back before pill break and bleed. Alternatively use an oestrogen-dominant pill e.g. Cilest®. (⚠ avoid in focal migraine).

## Advice for patients: Patient experiences of migraine

'I get a terrible pain on one side of my head, with nausea and a dreadful throbbing headache. I'm very lethargic, totally lose my appetite and generally feel unwell … I become very sensitive to noise, lights and smells – especially strong perfume, which I never wear. I don't vomit, but I do feel sick… My whole digestive system seems to close down.'

'An attack will often start with a feeling of stiffness in my neck and shoulders. This is followed by a period of slight confusion; being unable to find the right word in conversation, for example, or finding that I've typed absolute gobbledegook into my computer.'

'Sometimes, but not always, I experience visual disturbances which start with black flecks floating down in the outside corners of my vision. These can progress to blind spots in my vision, sometimes surrounded by brightly coloured zigzag lines. I also become extremely sensitive to light and I need to wear sunglasses, even on a dull day.'

'The pain starts as a dull ache in my left temple, quickly progressing to a pulsating throb that engulfs the whole left side of my head, face and neck. This is overscored by sharp shooting pains from the back of my neck to my eye, as if someone is drilling through from my neck and out into my eye. Everyday noises, such as the ticking of a clock, seem deafeningly loud. I then start to feel nauseous with a bad taste in my mouth and I become extremely sensitive to smells, even normal things such as coffee and paper. Smells such as paint, diesel or perfume are unbearable and can make me vomit.'

'The nausea often leads to vomiting, so even water won't stay down. Sometimes the vomiting is accompanied by diarrhoea.'

### Information and support
**Migraine Action Association** ☎ 0116 275 8317 🖳 www.migraine.org.uk
**The Migraine Trust** ☎ 020 7462 6601 🖳 www.migrainetrust.org

## Further information:

**British Association for the Study of Headache** Guidelines for all doctors in the diagnosis and management of migraine and tension-type headache (2007) 🖳 www.bash.org.uk

# Other headaches

**Assessment and differential diagnosis of headache:** 📖 pp.52–3

**Chronic daily headache:** Prevalence 4%. Defined as any headache that occurs > 15d./mo. Treat the cause. *Common causes:*

- Tension headache (below)
- Cervicogenic headache
- Medication overuse headache (below)
- Migraine
- Errors of refraction (usually mild, frontal and in the eyes themselves, and absent on waking).

**Tension-type headache:** Associated with stress and anxiety and/or functional or structural abnormalities of the head or neck. Prevalence ≈2%. ♀:♂≈2:1. Symptoms begin aged <10y. in 15% patients. Prevalence ↓ with age. Family history of similar headaches is common (40%) but twin studies do not suggest a genetic basis. Distinguish between episodic and chronic tension-type headache:

- *Episodic:* Defined as headache lasting 30min. to 7d. and occurring <180d./y. (<15d./mo.)
- *Chronic:* Headaches on ≥15d./mo (≥180d./y.) for ≥6mo.

In both cases, pain:

- Is bilateral, pressing, and/or tightening in quality
- Of mild or moderate intensity
- Does not prohibit activities
- Is not aggravated by routine physical activity
- Is not associated with vomiting
- Is associated with ≥1 of: nausea, photophobia, or phonophobia

**Management:**

- Reassure of no serious underlying pathology
- Try measures to alleviate stress – relaxation; massage; yoga; exercise. Cognitive therapy is probably effective but not widely available[CE].
- Treat musculoskeletal symptoms with physiotherapy.

*Drug therapy:* Analgesics are of limited value and might make matters worse (see medication overuse headache).

- *Headache <2x/wk:* Simple analgesia e.g. paracetamol, ibuprofen. Avoid codeine-containing preparations.
- *Chronic headache:* Amitriptyline 25–75mg nocte may help. Stop once improvement maintained for >4–6mo.

**Medication overuse (analgesic) headache:** Persistent headache may develop in patients with other causes of headache e.g. tension headache or migraine if they overuse the medication used to treat those conditions. Implicated drugs include: ergotamine, triptans, aspirin, paracetamol and NSAIDs. ♀:♂≈3:1. Ask any patient complaining of chronic daily headache to give a detailed account of medication use (including OTC) – a diary can be helpful.

**Management:** Aim for the patient to withdraw from the overused medication. Warn that symptoms may worsen initially (days 3–7) before improving.

**Cluster headaches (migrainous neuralgia):** Clusters of extremely painful headaches focused around 1 eye with associated autonomic symptoms (drooping eyelid, red watery eye, runny or blocked nose). May occur at any age but rare <20y. ♂:♀≈6:1. More common in smokers. Pain lasts up to 1h. and occurs 1–2x/d. every day for 4–12wk. then disappears for 1–2y. Recurrences affect the same side. Onset is often predictable (1–2h. after falling asleep; after alcohol).

**Management:** Refer for specialist advice. *Drug treatments:*

*Acute attack:*
- 100% oxygen at a rate of 7–12l/min.
- 5-HT$_1$ agonists e.g. sumatriptan (6mg s/cut) – stop 75% attacks in <15min.

*Prophylaxis:* Consider if attacks are frequent, last >3wk. or cannot be treated effectively. *Options:*
- Verapamil (unlicensed) – stops 66% attacks.
- Lithium (unlicensed) – used as for manic depression.
- Prednisolone 60–100mg od for 2–5l with rapid tapering over 2–3 wk.
- Ergotamine (unlicensed) – taken ½ h. before the attack is due. Should not be used for prolonged periods.
- Methysergide – effective but use limited by side effects. Only used if other drugs are contraindicated, not tolerated, or ineffective.

**Temporal arteritis:** Unilateral throbbing headache, facial pain, scalp tenderness e.g. on brushing hair, and/or jaw claudication. Visual symptoms – amaurosis fugax, diplopia, sudden loss of vision/blindness.
- ***Blood:*** ↑ ESR (usually >30) ± normocytic anaemia.
- ***Temporal artery biopsy:*** Refer urgently. Biopsy may be –ve even in true cases due to skip lesions. Do not withhold treatment whilst awaiting biopsy – but if steroids ≥2wk. +ve biopsy is less likely.

**Management:** Prescribe prednisolone 1mg/kg/d. (maximum 60mg od.); refer urgently to ophthalmology.
- In all cases, ↓ dose of prednisolone as symptoms allow e.g. by 2.5mg every 4wk. until taking 10mg prednisolone od, then by 1mg/mo. to 5mg od, then more slowly. Check ESR with dose changes. Stop steroid reduction and recheck ESR if ↑ symptoms. At the start of treatment give osteoporosis prophylaxis and supply with a steroid card (□ pp.102–3).
- Most patients require >2y. of treatment. Relapse is common after stopping treatment (50% if stopped after 2y.). Review diagnosis.

**GP Notes:**

ⓘ >1 type of headache may co-exist—consider each separately.

**Advice for patients: Information and support**

Organization for the understanding of cluster headaches (OUCH UK) ☎ 01646 651 979 🖥 www.ouchuk.org

**Further information:**
British Association for the Study of Headache Guidelines for all doctors in the diagnosis and management of migraine and tension type headache (2007) 🖥 www.bash.org.uk

# Trigeminal neuralgia, post-herpetic neuralgia and diabetic neuropathy pain

**Trigeminal neuralgia:**
- Paroxysms of intense stabbing, burning or 'electric shock' type pain lasting seconds to minutes in the trigeminal (V) nerve distribution.
- 96% unilateral.
- Mandibular/maxillary > ophthalmic division.
- Between attacks there are no symptoms.
- Frequency of attacks is highly variable ranging from hundreds of attacks/d. to remissions lasting years.
- Pain is often provoked by movement of the face (talking, eating, laughing) or by touching the skin (shaving, washing).
- Can occur at any age but more common >50y. ♀>♂.
- Unknown cause. More common in patients with MS and ♀ with ↑BP.

**Management:** Spontaneous remission may occur.
- Carbamazepine to ↓ frequency and intensity of attacks. NNT=1.8[C]. Start at low dose e.g. 100mg od/bd and ↑ dose over a period of weeks until symptoms are controlled. Usual dose ≈200mg tds. Oxcarbazine is an alternaive
- Gabapentin to ↓ frequency and intensity of attacks. Start with 300mg od on day 1. On day 2 ↑ to 300mg bd and ↑ again to 300mg tds on day 3. Increase further according to response, to a maximum of 1.8g daily (in divided doses). Pregabalin may also be used, up to 300mg/d in divided doses.

*Refer to neurology if:*
- <50y. old
- Neurological deficit between attacks
- If treatment with carbamazepine/gabapentin fails – specialist options include lamotrigine, duloxetine, baclofen or phenytoin, or surgical intervention.

**Post-herpetic neuralgia:** Herpes zoster (shingles) affects up to 50% of all people who live to 85y. Its most common complication is post-herpetic neuralgia – pain which persists months or years after the rash has healed.

**Definitions:**
- Acute herpetic neuralgia – <30d. after rash onset (61% >60y.)
- Subacute herpetic neuralgia – 30–120d. after rash onset (24% >60y.)
- Postherpetic neuralgia – pain lasting ≥120d. from rash onset (13% >60y. at 6mo.; 2% after 5y.)

**Risk factors:** Risk factors are cumulative. If all three are present, risk of persisting pain 6mo. after rash onset ~50–75%.
- ↑ age (especially >50y. –20% develop post-herpetic neuralgia following an acute attack of shingles if aged 60–65y.; 34% if aged >80y.)
- Severe attack of shingles with a lot of acute pain and/or severe rash
- Prodrome of dermatomal pain before onset of rash.

**Symptoms/signs:** Usually confined to the involved dermatome and include pain, increased sensitivity, itching, and paraesthesia. There is usually nothing to find on examination.

## Management:

*Prevention* – treatment of the acute shingles infection with antivirals e.g. aciclovir, famciclovir or valaciclovir ↓ duration of acute symptoms but does not ↓ risk of post-herpetic neuralgia. Treatment must be initiated early (i.e. <2d. after onset of symptoms). More likely to be cost and risk efficient in patients >50y.

*Treatment:*
- Tricyclic antidepressants: NNT = 2.2[C] – e.g. amitriptyline 25mg nocte – ↑ dose in steps of 25mg until pain relief is achieved (usual dose ≈75mg nocte). Start at lower dose (e.g. 10mg) and ↑ in smaller steps (e.g. 10mg) if elderly/frail.
- Anticonvulsants: Carbamazepine and gabapentin (NNT=3.9)[C] are both effective – use as for trigeminal neuralgia.
- Other measures: Capsaicin cream, topical LA (e.g. lidocaine patches), opioids e.g. tramadol, morphine, oxycodone.
- If not succeeding in controlling pain, and pain is having a significant effect on quality of life, refer to the pain clinic.

**Painful diabetic neuropathy:** Painful diabetic neuropathy is likely to develop when glucose control is poor.

## Management:
- Optimize blood sugar control.
- Give paracetamol, tramadol and/or NSAID for mild/moderate pain.
- If ineffective, consider treatment with a tricyclic antidepressant (NNT = 1.3[C] e.g. amitriptyline – use as for post-herpetic neuralgia), an anticonvulsant (e.g. carbamazepine – NNT = 2.3; gabapentin – NNT = 3.8; phenytoin – NNT = 2.1 – dosage is as for trigeminal neuralgia) or opioid (e.g. oxycodone – NNT = 2.6).
- Topical agents e.g. Capsaicin cream may also be helpful.
- If not succeeding in pain control, refer to the pain clinic or endocrinologist managing the patient's DM.

## Further information:

**BMJ** ▣ www.bmj.com
- Merrison and Fuller. Treatment options for trigeminal neuralgia. (2003) **327:** 1360–1.

## Cochrane Reviews
- Wiffen *et al.* Anticonvulsant drugs for acute and chronic pain
- Saarto and Wiffen. Antidepressants for neuropathic pain
- Wiffen *et al.* Carbamazepine for acute and chronic pain
- Wiffen *et al.* Gabapentin for acute and chronic pain
- Li *et al.* Antiviral treatment for preventing post-herpetic neuralgia.

---

### Advice for patients: Information and support

**Neuropathy Trust** ▣ www.neurocentre.com
**Trigeminal Neuralgia Association UK** ☎ 01883 370214
▣ www.tna.org.uk
**Diabetes UK** ☎ 0845 120 2960 ▣ www.diabetes.org.uk

# Low back pain

## Definitions:
- *Acute low back pain:* New episode of low back pain of <6wk. duration. Common – lifetime prevalence 58%
- *Chronic low back pain:* Back pain lasting >3mo. If present >1y. → poor prognosis

## Causes of back pain: Table 3.3

## Prevention of back pain:
- Regular exercise
- Optimize weight
- Advice on posture, working environment and lifting techniques
- Correct uneven leg length of >2–3cm measured from pubis to medial malleolus

## History:

### ASK:
- Circumstances of pain – history of injury; duration
- Nature and severity of pain – pain/stiffness mainly at rest or at night, easing with movement suggests inflammation e.g. discitis, spondyloarthropathy
- Associated symptoms e.g. numbness, weakness, bowel or bladder symptoms
- PMH—past illnesses (e.g. carcinoma), previous back problems
- Exclude pain not coming from the back (e.g. GI or GU pain)

## Examination:
- Deformity e.g. kyphosis (typical of ankylosing spondylitis), loss of lumbar lordosis (common in acute mechanical back pain), scoliosis.
- Palpate for tenderness, step deformity, and muscle spasm.
- Assess flexion, extension, lateral flexion, and rotation of the back whilst standing.
- Ask to lie down – this gives a good indication of how severe severity of symptoms are.
- In lower limbs, look for muscle wasting and check power, sensory loss and reflexes (knee jerk and ankle jerk). Assess straight leg raise (SLR) – sciatica is present if SLR on one side elicits back/buttock pain (usually ipsilateral but can be either side) compared with SLR on the other side.

| ⚠ 'Red flags': | |
|---|---|
| - <20 or >55y. | - Immune suppression |
| - Non-mechanical pain | - IV drug use |
| - Pain that worsens when supine | - Taking steroids |
| - Night-time pain | - Unwell |
| - Thoracic pain | - Weight ↓ |
| - Past history of carcinoma | - Widespread neurology |
| - Human immunodeficiency virus (HIV) | - Structural deformity |

**Management of acute pain in the community:** Triage according to history and examination – Figure 3.1, 📖 p.65.

**Table 3.3 Causes of back pain: age suggests the most likely cause**

| Age (y.) | Causes | |
|---|---|---|
| 15–30 | • Postural<br>• Mechanical<br>• Prolapsed disc<br>• Trauma | • Fracture<br>• Ankylosing spondylosis<br>• Spondylolisthesis<br>• Pregnancy |
| 30–50 | • Postural<br>• Degenerative joint disease<br>• Prolapsed disc | • Discitis<br>• Spondyloarthropathies |
| >50 | • Postural<br>• Degenerative<br>• Osteoporotic collapse<br>• Paget's disease | • Malignancy (lung, breast, prostate, thyroid, kidney)<br>• Myeloma |
| Other causes | • Referred pain<br>• Spinal stenosis | • Cauda equina tumours<br>• Spinal infection |

**Table 3.4 Neurology associated with lumbosacral nerve root entrapment**

| Root | Sensory changes | Motor weakness | Reflex changes |
|---|---|---|---|
| L2 | Front of thigh | Hip flexion/adduction | None |
| L3 | Inner thigh | Knee extension | Knee |
| L4 | Inner shin | Knee extension<br>Foot dorsiflexion | Knee |
| L5 | Outer shin<br>Dorsum of foot | Knee flexion<br>Foot inversion<br>Big toe dorsiflexion | None |
| S1 | Lateral side of foot/sole | Knee flexion<br>Foot plantarflexion | Ankle |

63

**GP Notes: Questions to ask when assessing low back pain**

P What factors Provoke and Palliate the pain?
Q What type or Quality of pain is it?
R Does the pain Radiate anywhere?
S How Severe is the pain and are there any Systemic symptoms?
T At what Times is the pain at its best/worst?

**Advice for patients: Information and support**

The Back Book. HMSO ISBN 0017020788
Arthritis Research Campaign ☎ 0870 8505000 🖥 www.arc.org.uk

The 'PQRST' rule is reproduced with permission from the *ABC of Rheumatology*, BMJ Publishing Group.

**❶ Do not X-ray routinely:** X-rays require a high radiation dose and +ve findings are rare. *Exceptions:* no improvement in >6 wk.; young (< 25y.) – X-ray SI joints to exclude ankylosing spondylitis; elderly – to exclude vertebral collapse/ malignancy; history of trauma; 'red flag' signs
*For patients who do not require immediate referral:*

- *Explain the likely natural history* of the pain and advise to avoid bed rest and try to maintain normal activities (↓ chance of chronic pain).
- *Prescribe analgesia* e.g. paracetamol ± NSAIDs and suggest self-help exercises.
- *Consider referral for physiotherapy, chiropractic or osteopathy –* Refer patients with nerve root irritation or simple backache not returning to normal activities by 6wk. for back exercises (if available locally) or physiotherapy, chiropractic or osteopathy. Refer sooner if in a lot of pain. Do not refer if there is any possible serious pathology.

---

**Cauda equina syndrome:** Results from compression of the cauda equina below L2 e.g. by disc protrusion at L4/5. Presents with:
- Numbness of the buttocks and backs of thighs
- Urinary/faecal incontinence
- Lower motor neurone weakness - signs depend on level at which the cauda equine is compressed:
  - L4 – loss of dorsiflexion of the foot (and toes – L4/5)
  - S1 – loss of ankle reflex, plantarflexion and eversion of the foot

**Management:** Refer/admit as a neurological emergency. Rapid surgical intervention increases the chance of full motor and sphincter recovery.

---

**Back pain and malignancy:** 📖 p.149.

**Risk factors for developing chronic pain/long-term disability:**
- Belief that pain and activity are harmful
- Sickness behaviours such as extended rest
- Social withdrawal
- Emotional problems e.g. low/negative mood, depression, anxiety, stress
- Problems with claims or compensation or time off work
- Overprotective family *or* lack of support
- Inappropriate expectations of treatment, e.g. low expectations of active participation in treatment

**Management of chronic pain:** Aim to help patients accept and cope with pain and to lead as full a life as possible. Education, exercise, and psychological approaches may ↓ disability.

- *Exclude spinal pathology and lesions amenable to surgery* e.g. disc protrusion and spondylolisthesis.
- *Consider referral to a pain clinic.*
- *Analgesics* can help sleep disturbance but are of limited benefit if used regularly in the long term. Reserve for exacerbations.
- *Tricyclic antidepressants* e.g. amitriptyline 25–75mg nocte may help.
- *Other approaches* – Back supports (e.g. corsets or belts); heel raises (to correct uneven leg length) and TENS are sometimes helpful.

**Further information:**
NICE Low back pain (2009) 🖥 www.nice.org.uk

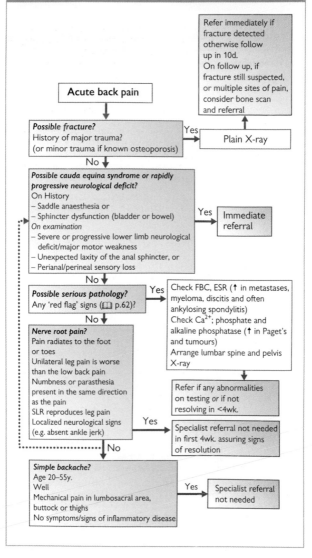

**Figure 3.1 Triage of acute back pain**

**Acute back pain**

*Possible fracture?*
History of major trauma?
(or minor trauma if known osteoporosis) → **Yes** → Plain X-ray → Refer immediately if fracture detected otherwise follow up in 10d.
On follow up, if fracture still suspected, or multiple sites of pain, consider bone scan and referral

No ↓

*Possible cauda equina syndrome or rapidly progressive neurological deficit?*
On History
– Saddle anaesthesia or
– Sphincter dysfunction (bladder or bowel)
On examination
– Severe or progressive lower limb neurological deficit/major motor weakness
– Unexpected laxity of the anal sphincter, or
– Perianal/perineal sensory loss → **Yes** → Immediate referral

No ↓

*Possible serious pathology?*
Any 'red flag' signs (☐ p.62)? → **Yes** → Check FBC, ESR (↑ in metastases, myeloma, discitis and often ankylosing spondylitis)
Check Ca²⁺; phosphate and alkaline phosphatase (↑ in Paget's and tumours)
Arrange lumbar spine and pelvis X-ray → Refer if any abnormalities on testing *or* if not resolving in <4wk.

No ↓

*Nerve root pain?*
Pain radiates to the foot or toes
Unilateral leg pain is worse than the low back pain
Numbness or parasthesia present in the same direction as the pain
SLR reproduces leg pain
Localized neurological signs (e.g. absent ankle jerk) → **Yes** → Specialist referral not needed in first 4wk. assuring signs of resolution

No ↓

*Simple backache?*
Age 20–55y.
Well
Mechanical pain in lumbosacral area, buttock or thighs
No symptoms/signs of inflammatory disease → **Yes** → Specialist referral not needed

### 1. Stretching exercises

NB. Upper knee should be directly above lower knee

**1. Back stretch (stretches back muscles)** Lie on your back, hands above your head. Bend your knees and, keeping your feet on the floor, roll your knees to one side, slowly. Stay on one side for 10 seconds. **Repeat 3 times each side**.

 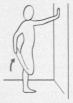

**2. Deep lunge (stretches muscles in front of thigh and abdomen)** Kneel on one knee, the other foot in front. Lift the knee up; keep looking forwards. Hold for 5 seconds and **repeat 3 times each side**.

**3. One-leg stand—front (stretches front thigh)** Steady yourself with one hand on something for support. Bend one leg up behind you. Hold your foot for 10 seconds and **repeat 3 times each side**.

 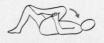

**4. One-leg stand—back (stretches muscles at back of leg)** Steady yourself, then put one leg, straight, up on a chair. Bend the other knee in to stretch the hamstrings. **Repeat 3 times each side**.

**5. Knee to chest (stretches muscles of bottom—gluteals)** Lie on your back. Bring one knee up and pull it gently into your chest for 5 seconds. **Repeat for up to 5 times each side**.

## 2. Strength, stamina and stabilizing exercises

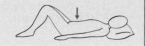

**1. Pelvic tilt** Lie down with your knees bent. Tighten your stomach muscles, flattening your back against the floor. Hold for 5 seconds. **Repeat 5 times**.

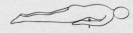

**2. Stomach tone ('transverse tummy')** Lie on your front with your arms by your side, head on one side. Pull in your stomach muscles, centred around your tummy button. Hold for 5 seconds. **Repeat 3 times**. Build up to 10 seconds and repeat during the day, while walking or standing. Keep breathing during this exercise.

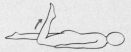

**3. Buttock tone (gluteals)** Bend one leg up behind you while lying on your front. Then lift your bent knee just off the floor. Hold for up to 8 seconds. **Repeat 5 times each side**.

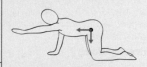

**4. Deep stomach muscle tone (stabilizes lower back)** Kneel on all fours with a small curve in your lower back. Let your stomach relax completely. Pull the lower part of your stomach upwards so that you lift your back (without arching it) away from the floor. Hold for 10 seconds. Keep breathing! **Repeat 10 times**.

**5. Back stabilizer** Kneel on all fours with your back straight. Tighten your stomach. Keeping your back in position, raise one arm in front of you and hold for 10 seconds. Try to keep your pelvis level and do not rotate your body. **Repeat 10 times each side**. To progress, try lifting one leg behind you instead of your arm.

Exercises on these pages are reproduced with permission of the Arthritis and Rheumatism Campaign 🖳 www.arc.org.uk

# Osteoarthritis (OA) pain

Osteoarthritis (OA) is the most important cause of locomotor disability. It used to be considered 'wear and tear' of the bone/cartilage of synovial joints but is now recognized as a metabolically active process involving the whole joint — i.e. cartilage, bone, synovium, capsule and muscle.

The main reason for patients seeking medical help is pain. Level of pain and disability are greatly influenced by the patient's personality, anxiety, depression and activity, and often do not correlate well with clinical signs.

**Risk factors:** ↑ age (uncommon <45y.); ♀>♂; ↑ in black and Asian populations; genetic predisposition; obesity; abnormal mechanical loading of joint e.g. instability; poor muscle function; post-meniscectomy; certain occupations e.g. farming.

**Symptoms and signs:** Joint pain ± stiffness, synovial thickening, deformity, effusion, crepitus, muscle weakness and wasting and ↓ function. Most commonly affects hip, knee and base of thumb. Typically exacerbations occur that may last weeks to months. Nodal OA, with swelling of the distal interphalageal joints (Heberdens nodes) has a familial tendency.

**Investigations:** X-rays may show ↓ joint space, cysts and sclerosis in subchondral bone, and osteophytes. OA is common and may be a coincidental finding. Exclude other causes of pain e.g. check FBC and ESR if inflammatory arthritis is suspected (normal or mildly ↑ in OA — ESR >30 suggests RA or psoriatic arthritis).

**Management of osteoarthritis in primary care:** Employ a holistic approach. Assess affect of OA on the patient's functioning, quality of life, occupation, mood, relationships and leisure activities. Formulate a management plan with the patient that includes self-management strategies, effects of co-morbidities and regular review.

*Information and advice:* Give information and advice on all relevant aspects of osteoarthritis and its management. The arc website (⌨ www.arc.org.uk) has a wide range of information leaflets for patients. Use the whole multidisciplinary team e.g. refer to
- Physiotherapist for advice on exercises, strapping and splints
- OT for aids
- Chiropodist for foot care and insoles
- Social worker for advice on disability benefits and housing
- Orthopaedics for surgery if significant disability/night pain.

*↓ load on the joint:* Weight reduction can ↓ symptoms and may ↓ progression in knee OA. Using a walking stick in the opposite hand to the affected hip and cushioned insoles/shoes (e.g. trainers) can also help.

*Exercise and improving muscle strength:* ↓ pain and disability e.g. walking (for OA knee), swimming (for OA back and hip but may make neck worse), cycling (for OA knee but may worsen patellofemoral OA). Refer to physiotherapy for advice on exercises especially isometric exercises for the less mobile.

*Pain control:*
- Use non pharmacological methods first (activity, exercise, weight ↓, footwear modification, walking stick, TENS, local heat/cold treatments).
- Regular paracetamol (1g qds) is first-line drug treatment for all OA and/or topical NSAIDS for knee/hand OA only. Topical NSAIDs have less side effects than oral NSAIDs and are more acceptable to patients.
- Use opioids, oral NSAIDs or COX2 inhibitors as second line agents in addition to, or instead of paracetamol. Use the lowest effective dose for the shortest possible time. Co-prescribe a proton pump inhibitor (e.g. omeprazole 20mg od) with NSAIDs and COX2 inhibitors.
- Low dose antidepressants e.g. amitriptyline 10–75mg nocte (unlicensed) are a useful adjunct especially for pain causing sleep disturbance.
- Capsaicin cream can also be helpful for knee/hand OA. NICE does not recommend rubefacients for other OA

***Aspiration of joint effusions and joint injections:*** Can help in exacerbations. Some patients respond well to long-acting steroid injections - it may be worth considering a trial of a single treatment. Hyaluronic acid knee injections are not recommended by NICE.

***Complementary therapies:*** ~60% of sufferers from OA are thought to use CAM e.g. copper bracelets, acupuncture, food supplements, dietary manipulation. There is good evidence chiropractic/osteopathy can be helpful for back pain, but otherwise evidence of effectiveness is scanty. Advise patients to find a reputable practitioner with accredited training who is a member of a recognised professional body and carries professional indemnity insurance.

***Glucosamine:*** ☞ It is controversial whether glucosamine modifies OA progression. NICE does not recommend prescription of glucosamine but patients may wish to purchase it over-the-counter.

***Psychological factors:*** Have a major impact on the disability from OA. Education about the disease, and emphasis that it is not progressive in most people, is important. Seek and treat depression and anxiety with screening tools.

## Refer:
- ***To rheumatology*** to confirm diagnosis if co-existent psoriasis (psoriatic arthritis mimics OA and can be missed by radiologists); rule out 2° causes of OA (e.g. pseudogout, haemochromatosis) if young OA or odd distribution; if joint injection is thought worthwhile but you lack expertise or confidence to do it.
- ***To orthopaedics:*** if symptoms are severe for joint replacement. Refer as an emergency if you suspect joint sepsis.

## Further information:
**NICE** Osteoarthritis: the care and management of osteoarthritis in adults (2008) www.nice.org.uk
**Bandolier** Topical NSAIDs (2003)
🖥 www.jr2.ox.ac.uk/bandolier/band110/b110-6.html

## Information and support for patients:
**Arthritis Research Campaign (arc)** ☎0870 8505000 🖥 www.arc.org.uk

# Providing joint and soft tissue injections

Steroids can have a potent local anti-inflammatory effect and dramatically improve certain musculoskeletal problems. Most joint injections are straightforward and can be undertaken within a general practice setting.

## Preparation for the procedure:
- Take a history, make a careful examination and have a clear diagnosis before considering injecting steroids.
- Gather the needles, syringes, a sterile container (for sending aspirated fluid to the laboratory), steroid, local anaesthetic, skin preparation fluid (e.g. chlorhexidine), cotton wool and elastoplast beforehand.
- The injected joint should be rested for 2–3d. afterwards if possible – certainly heavy activity should be avoided. Make sure the patient is comfortable, has given informed consent and knows what to expect.

**Consent:** Patient consent for the procedure must be sought and recorded in the notes. This involves giving enough information about the procedure and other possible treatment options to allow the patient to make an informed decision about whether to proceed. The patient and consenting doctor should then both sign the consent form. The form should be filed in the patient's medical records.

ⓘ Part of the specification for a directed enhanced service for minor surgery includes the use of a standard NHS consent form available via the Department of Health website (🖥 www.dh.gov.uk).

**Steroid preparations:** (↑ order of potency) – hydrocortisone acetate, methylprednisolone acetate, triamcinolone hexacetonide.

**Local anaesthetic (LA):** e.g. lidocaine 1% can be mixed with the steroid for some injections – a local anaesthetic effect occurs immediately and lasts 2–4h. The patient may then experience some return of symptoms (pain) before the steroid takes effect – warn the patient of this possibility.

## Follow up:
- Some injections are painful at administration – this is normal for tennis elbow and plantar faciitis.
- Severe or increasing pain ~48h. after injection may indicate sepsis – advise the patient to return urgently if this occurs.
- If steroid is injected close to the skin surface (as in tennis elbow), skin dimpling and pigment loss can occur – warn the patient.

⚠ Never attempt a procedure if you are unsure about it – know the boundaries of your experience and abilities.

- Always use aseptic technique.
- Do not inject if there is local sepsis (e.g. cellulitis) or any possibility of joint infection.
- Never inject into the substance of a tendon – this may cause rupture (in tenosynovitis, steroid is injected into the tendon sheath).
- Injections should not require pressure on the syringe plunger – if so, the needle is probably not correctly located (tennis elbow is an exception).
- Undertake as few injections as possible to settle the problem – often, 1 is sufficient. If no improvement after 2–3 injections then reconsider the diagnosis.
- Do no more than 3–4 injections/patient/appointment and no more than 3–4 in any single joint/year – more than this ↑ risk of systemic absorption and joint damage.

**Advice for patients: Information and support**

Arthritis Research Campaign (ARC) Patient information leaflet: local steroid injections ☎ 0870 850 5000 🖥 www.arc.org.uk

**GMS Contract**

Minor surgery can be provided as an additional service or directed enhanced service (📖 p.264).

**Further information:**

**Silver T**. *Joint and soft tissue injection: injecting with confidence* (2001). Radcliffe Medical Press ISBN: 1857755642.

❗ Most hospital rheumatology departments have a joint injection clinic and are happy to allow GPs to watch to gain experience.

# Lower limb injections

**The knee:** Joint effusions are common (e.g. trauma, ligament strains, OA, RA, gout). Aspiration of fluid can:
- Help make a diagnosis e.g. gout
- Be a therapeutic procedure – draining a tense effusion can relieve pain
- Precede administration of steroids e.g. RA flare

Aspirated fluid should be clear or slightly yellow and not purulent. If aspirating an effusion, send the fluid for analysis.

> ⚠ Any sign of infection within the joint prohibits steroid use.

### Technique for aspiration and joint injection:
- Lie the patient on a couch with their knee slightly bent – place a pillow under the knee as this relaxes the muscles.
- Palpate the joint space under the lateral or medial edge of the patella and inject/aspirate just below the superior border of the patella with the needle horizontal – Figure 3.2.
- Use a green (21-gauge) needle.
- If aspirating and then injecting steroids, maintain the needle in position and swap the syringe.
- Normal doses of steroid are triamcinolone 20mg or methylprednisolone 40mg.
- In prepatella bursitis, aspiration and injection of hydrocortisone 25mg into the bursa can help settle inflammation.

**Plantar fasciitis:** Painful area in the middle of the heel pad can be helped by steroid injection into the most tender spot – this hurts so advise analgesia. Mixing lidocaine 1% with the steroid (e.g. triamcinolone 10–20mg) can help.

**Technique:** Two methods are commonly used (Figure 3.3):
- Injection through the tough skin of the sole of the foot (more accurate)
- Lateral approach (less painful)

Rest the foot for several days and use an inshoe heel pad. Rupture of the plantar fascia is a rare complication.

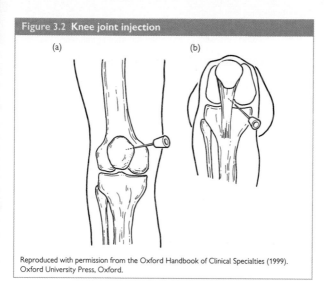

**Figure 3.2 Knee joint injection**

(a)    (b)

Reproduced with permission from the Oxford Handbook of Clinical Specialties (1999). Oxford University Press, Oxford.

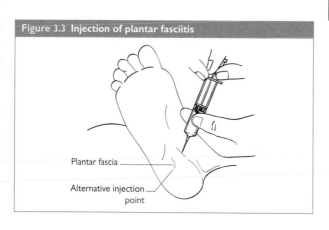

**Figure 3.3 Injection of plantar fasciitis**

Plantar fascia

Alternative injection point

# Upper limb injections

**Tenosynovitis:** Causes pain and stiffness in the line of the tendon, and crepitus over the affected tendon. The most common site is the base of the thumb (DeQuervain's tenosynovitis).

Injecting steroid and local anaesthetic (e.g. hydrocortisone 25mg and 1ml 1% lignocaine) into the space between the tendon and the sheath can help.

## Technique:
- Insert the needle along the line of the tendon just distal to the point of maximum tenderness.
- Advance the needle proximally into the tendon (felt as a resistance) and then slowly withdraw until the resistance disappears. The tip of the needle is now in the tendon sheath.
- It is now safe to inject – the tendon sheath may swell.
- Advise the patient to rest the affected area for several days and avoid the precipitating activity.

**Carpal tunnel syndrome:** Can be relieved by steroid injection.

## Technique:
- Sit the patient with their hand resting on a firm surface, palm up. The palmaris longus tendon can be seen by wrist flexion against resistance.
- Insert the needle at the distal skin crease, at 45° to the horizontal, pointing towards the fingers, Figure 3.4. just ulnar (little finger-side) to the palmaris tendon.
- Use a green (21-gauge) needle and advance it to about half its length. If there is sudden pain in the fingers you have hit the median nerve – withdraw the needle and reposition it.
- Inject steroid e.g. 10mg triamcinolone – if there is resistance the needle is not in the right place. Do not use LA as it causes finger numbness.
- Advise the patient to rest the hand for several days afterwards.

🛈 Palmaris longus is absent in 10% of individuals – inject between the tendons of flexor digitorum superficialis and flexor carpi radialis.

**Elbow:** Tennis or golfer's elbow respond well to steroid injection. Steroid is infiltrated into the tender spots at the tendon insertion rather than into a joint space. Thus, there is resistance on injection and it can be quite painful – warn the patient.

## Technique:
- Sit the patient with the elbow flexed to 90° and palpate the most tender spot.
- Insert the needle into that spot and inject 0.1–0.2ml of steroid (e.g. hydrocortisone 25mg/1ml). Then, without making a new skin puncture, move the needle in a fan shape around the area injecting small amounts of steroid – try to inject all the tender area. The steroid is injected relatively superficially so warn the patient about the possibility of skin dimpling or pigment loss.
- Pain of injection may last 48h. – advise resting the arm and taking analgesic medications.

🛈 A recent RCT showed that for Tennis elbow, steroid injection has significantly better effects in the short term (~6wk.) but poorer outcome long term compared to physiotherapy.

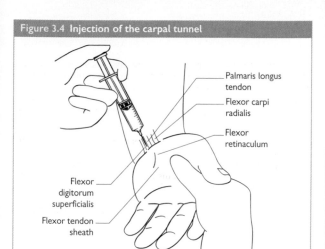

### Figure 3.4 Injection of the carpal tunnel

Palmaris longus tendon

Flexor carpi radialis

Flexor retinaculum

Flexor digitorum superficialis

Flexor tendon sheath

⚠ Pain may worsen after injection for up to 48h. before it improves – warn the patient of this possibility.

## Further information:

**BMJ** Bisset et al., Mobilisation with movement and exercise, corticosteroid injection, or wait and see for tennis elbow: randomised trial (2006) **333: 939** 🖳 www.bmj.com.

**Shoulder:** Injection can help rotator cuff problems, frozen shoulder, subacromial bursitis and rheumatoid arthritis. Injection can be located into either the shoulder joint or the subacromial space (Figure 3.5). Use an anterior or posterior approach for shoulder joint injection and lateral approach for the subacromial space. The joint space only communicates with the subacromial space if there is a rotator cuff tear – in which case steroid will reach the whole joint whichever approach is used.

**Technique:** *Anterior approach:*
- Sit patient with their arm relaxed at their side and slightly externally rotated. Palpate the space between the head of humerus and the coracoid process.
- Insert the needle (green, 21 gauge) horizontally into that gap ensuring the needle is lateral to the coracoid process – Figure 3.5(a). The needle will need to be inserted for most of its length to reach the joint space.
- Typical dose is 1ml steroid e.g. triamcinolone 20mg + 1ml 1% lidocaine.
- There should be no/little resistance to injecting the fluid – if there is, the needle is wrongly positioned.

**Technique:** *Lateral approach to subacromial space:*
- Sit patient with arm hanging down to side.
- Palpate the postero-lateral corner of the acromion.
- Insert the needle horizontally into the space beneath the acromion – Figure 3.5(b).
- Use 5ml 0.5% marcaine + triamcinolone 20mg.

**AC joint injection:** Can help the pain of OA.

**Technique:**
- Palpate the joint space – the needle can be inserted anteriorly or superiorly – if you push the needle too far you may enter the shoulder joint – Figure 3.6(c).
- Small joint space means only 0.2–0.5ml can be injected.
- Use a blue (23 gauge) needle and do not add LA.

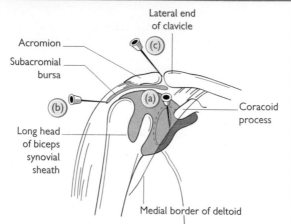

**Figure 3.5 Shoulder joint injection**

- Lateral end of clavicle
- Acromion
- Subacromial bursa
- (b)
- Long head of biceps synovial sheath
- (c)
- (a)
- Coracoid process
- Medial border of deltoid

(a) Anterior approach joint injection
(b) Subacromial space injection
(c) Acromioclavicular joint injection

Reproduced with modifications from the *Oxford Handbook of Clinical Specialties* (1999). Oxford University Press, Oxford.

# Chapter 4

# Principles of palliative care in general practice

# Palliative care

*'Any man's death diminishes me because I am involved in mankind'*
Devotions Meditation 17, John Donne 1572–1631.

**What is palliative care?** Palliative care starts when the emphasis changes from curing the patient and prolonging life to relieving symptoms and maintaining well-being or 'quality of life'.

**WHO definition:** 'Palliative care is an approach that improves the quality of life of patients and their families facing the problems associated with life-threatening illness, through the prevention and relief of suffering by means of early identification and impeccable assessment and treatment of pain and other problems, physical, psychosocial, and spiritual.'

**Features of palliative care:** Palliative care:
- Provides relief from pain and other distressing symptoms
- Affirms life and regards dying as a normal process
- Intends neither to hasten nor postpone death
- Focuses on enhancing quality of life, but may also positively influence the course of illness (though is not primarily concerned with producing long-term remission)
- Is person-, not disease-oriented
- Is holistic in nature
- Integrates the psychological and spiritual aspects of patient care
- Offers a support system to help patients live as actively as possible until death
- Offers a support system to help the family cope during the patient's illness and in their own bereavement
- Uses a multidisciplinary team approach to address the needs of patients and their families

**Who is palliative care appropriate for?** Many of us think of palliative care as being synonymous to care of patients dying with cancer. Palliative care is appropriate for *all* patients with active, progressive, far-advanced disease and not just patients with cancer – though the evidence base for the efficacy of interventions is largely based on experience with cancer patients.

**When should palliative care start?** Palliative care can be used in conjunction with other therapies that are intended to prolong life, such as chemotherapy or radiotherapy. It should dovetail into the ongoing active treatment of the patient's illness in the later stages of disease (Figure 4.1). It should not be withheld until all treatment alternatives for the underlying disease have been exhausted.

Figure 4.1 Model of active palliative care

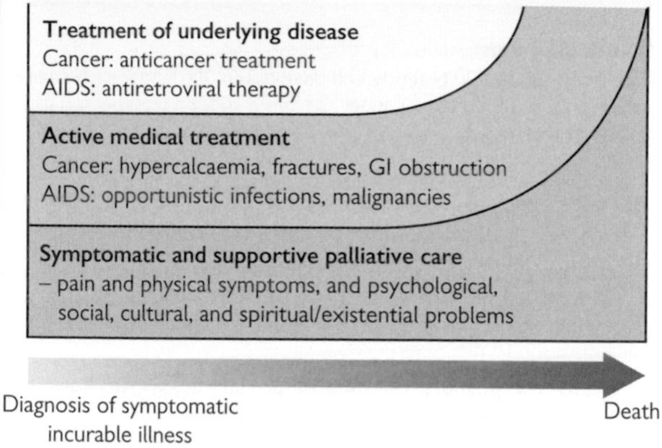

**Treatment of underlying disease**
Cancer: anticancer treatment
AIDS: antiretroviral therapy

**Active medical treatment**
Cancer: hypercalcaemia, fractures, GI obstruction
AIDS: opportunistic infections, malignancies

**Symptomatic and supportive palliative care**
– pain and physical symptoms, and psychological,
  social, cultural, and spiritual/existential problems

Diagnosis of symptomatic                                    Death
         incurable illness

Reproduced from Woodruff R. *Palliative Medicine*. 4th edition. Oxford University Press, (2004) with permission.

## Further information:

**WHO** Definition of palliative care
🖳 www.who.int/cancer/palliative/definition/en/
**Woodruff R** *Palliative Medicine*. (4th edition-2004). Oxford University Press ISBN: 019551677X
**NICE** Improving supportive and palliative care for adults with cancer. (2004). 🖳 www.nice.org.uk
**Watson et al.** *Oxford Handbook of Palliative Care*. (2005). Oxford University Press ISBN: 0198508972
**Woodruff and Doyle** *The IAHPC Manual of Palliative Care* (2nd Edition) (2004). IAHPC Press ISBN 0975852515
🖳 www.hospicecare.com/manual/IAHPCmanual.htm

# Palliative care in general practice

**Facts and figures:**
- The 'average' UK GP practice will have about 20 deaths each year of which only 5 will be from cancer, 2 from a sudden unexpected cause and the remaining 13 from chronic disease such as dementia, heart failure, and COPD.
- On average 47wk. of the final year of life are spent at home.
- GPs have 1–2 patients with terminal disease at any time and get more personally involved with them than any others.

**The challenge of palliative care in the community:** It is a sad fact that although most patients spend their final year of life at home, and would prefer to die at home, the majority are admitted to a hospital or institution to die.

**The role of the primary care team:** GPs and the primary care team have always been, and will continue to be, the main providers of palliative care for most patients but we often find palliative care difficult. Common concerns include:
- Not knowing enough about controlling symptoms
- Being reluctant to use powerful drugs in effective doses
- Worrying about the time commitment involved *and*
- Being afraid to expose oneself to painful emotions

**Problems encountered:** Problems arising in palliative care are a complex mix of physical, psychological, and social factors involving both patients and carers (Figure 4.2). To respond adequately, good lines of communication and close multidisciplinary teamwork is needed. Local palliative care teams are invaluable sources of advice and support and frequently produce booklets with advice on aspects of palliative care for GPs.

**The Gold Standards Framework:** Aims to improve the quality of palliative care provided by the primary care team by developing practice-based organization of care of dying patients. The framework focuses on:
- Optimizing continuity of care
- Teamwork
- Advanced planning (including out-of-hours cover)
- Symptom control
- Patient, carer, and staff support

Evaluation data show the framework ↑ the proportion of patients dying in their preferred place and improves quality of care as perceived by the practitioners involved.

**Additional qualifications:** Nationally, the 8wk., home study *Princess Alice Certificate in Essential Palliative Care* is held every 6mo. at sites across the UK. It has been endorsed by the *Gold Standards Framework*.

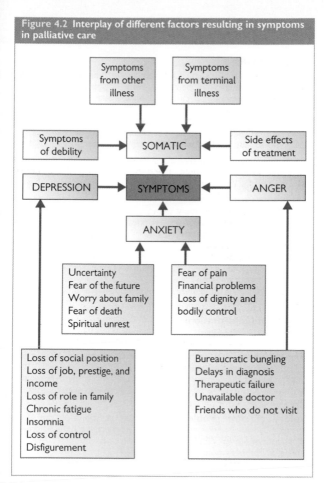

Figure 4.2 Interplay of different factors resulting in symptoms in palliative care

**Further information:**

**BMJ** Kenyon Z. *Palliative care in general practice* (1995) **311**: 888–9.
🖳 www.bmj.com
**Gold Standards Framework**
🖳 www.goldstandardsframework.nhs.uk
**Princess Alice Certificate in Essential Palliative Care** ☎ 01372 461845
E-mail: education@pah.org.uk
🖳 www.pah.org.uk/
**Hospice information** 🖳 www.helpthehospices.org.uk

# Assessment and planning action

### Role of the GP:
- GPs of patients receiving palliative care in the community are always team members – and may be the key workers who co-ordinate care.
- Maintain an open door policy and encourage patients and carers to seek help for problems early.
- Try to become familiar with a patient's disease. It is impossible to plan care without knowledge of the course and prognosis and an easy way to lose a patient's confidence if you appear ignorant of their condition.

### The setting:
- Wherever possible, meet the patient face-to-face. Avoid telephone discussions except for brief advice or when face-to-face meetings are not possible (e.g. if the patient is away and wants advice).
- Ensure privacy – turn your pager or mobile phone off if possible and ask reception staff not to interrupt.
- Sit down level with the patient.
- Allow enough time.
- Wherever possible, ensure the patient has a family member or friend with him/her for support.
- Use trained interpreters if the patient does not have sufficient English to communicate freely.

### Background information:
- *Introduce the discussion*—'We need to talk about your illness, the problems you have now and what we want to aim for.'
- *Find out what the patient and his/her family understand*—'Tell me what you know about your illness.'
- *Find out what they expect*—'What do you think is going to happen with your illness in the future?' *and/or* 'What do you want us to do for you?'

**Explore current problems:** Use open questions at the start, becoming directive when necessary – clarify, reflect, facilitate, listen.
- *Physical symptoms*—'Do you have any pain or discomfort?'; 'Are there any other symptoms that bother you?'
- *Psychological and/or spiritual symptoms*—'How are you coping in yourself?'
- *Social wellbeing*—'How are you coping at home?'; 'What do you do in the day?'; 'Do you need any help around the house?'
- *Wellbeing of the rest of the family*

Examine the patient as directed by the history.

**The benefits of listening:** Patients value being listened to because:
- They feel their problems have been understood
- It helps them to clarify or reframe their problems
- It helps them to feel an integral part of the care team
- It reassures them that they are not alone in their suffering
- They feel reassured that treatment is available and can help
- It helps them release pent-up feelings

## GP Notes:

**Interview style:** Problems are more likely to be identified where the doctor displays the following behaviours:

- Giving good eye contact from the start
- Clarifying presenting complaints
- Moving from open-ended to more closed questions
- Frequently making empathic remarks
- Being sensitive to verbal cues to emotional problems
- Being sensitive to non-verbal cues
- Avoiding reading or making notes (or computer entries)
- Controlling patients' overtalkativeness

### Checklist of areas to cover:

- Can physical symptoms be improved?
- Can the psychological symptoms be improved (including self-esteem)?
- Can spiritual symptoms be improved?
- Can functioning within the home be improved? (aids and adaptations within the home, extra help)
- Can functioning in the community be improved? (mobility outside the home, work, social activities)
- Can the patient's or carer's financial state be improved? (benefits)
- Does the carer/family need more support? (voluntary and self-help organizations, extra help, sitting service, respite care, counselling)

| GMS Contract | | | |
|---|---|---|---|
| Palliative care 3 | The practice has a complete register available of all patients in need of palliative care/support irrespective of age | 3 points | |
| Palliative care 2 | The practice has regular (at least 3-monthly) multidisciplinary case review meetings where all patients on the palliative care register are discussed | 3 points | |
| Cancer 1 | The practice can produce a record of all cancer patients diagnosed after 1.4.2003 | 5 points | |
| Cancer 3 | The % of patients with cancer diagnosed within the last 18mo. who have a patient review recorded as ocurring within 6mo. of the practice receiving confirmation of the diagnosis | up to 6 points | 40–90% |
| Education 7 | The practice has undertaken a minimum of 12 significant event reviews in the past 3y. which could include (if these have occurred) new cancer diagnoses | Total of 4 points for 12 significant event reviews | |

**Planning appropriate care:**

- Summarize the history back to the patient and give an opportunity for the patient to fill in any gaps.
- Draw up a problem list with the patient.
- What treatments can be offered? Discuss realistic possibilities in the context of the patient's and your view of the present and future. If agreement is not reached, interventions can be trialled for a specified time. Explain the possible benefits and burdens (or futility) of any intervention.
- Never say 'there is nothing more we can do'. There is always something more that can be done. Patients interpret a statement like this to mean there is no treatment for any further symptoms and both the patient and family feel abandoned. You can tell patients there is no further treatment for the underlying disease, but stress that you will still be providing continuing care and symptom control.
- Outline a management plan with the patient with provision that it could be modified should circumstances change. Shared decision-making between patient and doctor improves concordance and patient satisfaction as well as clinical outcome.
- Set a review date.

**Sharing medical information:**

- Give patients as much, or as little, information as they want – if unsure, ask them how much they want.
- Share information in a sympathetic way – not abruptly or bluntly.
- Give information in a way the patient can understand – speak clearly, avoid medical jargon and euphemisms.
- Ask patients to repeat back what they understand.
- Respond kindly to emotional outbursts.

**Discussing prognosis:** Avoid giving precise prognoses. Explain the uncertainty in estimating prognosis and give a realistic time range as this enables the patient to deal with their affairs and attend to family relationships.

**Discussing referral to the palliative care services:** Patients have variable experience of palliative care services. Some are terrified of referral as they see hospices as places to die and referral means to them that they are going to die – and soon. Others have more positive views – either through past experience when palliative care services have been involved with friends or relatives or because they have been involved in the hospice movement themselves e.g. as volunteers.

Introduce the possibility of referral to palliative care services when it becomes clear the patient is suffering from an incurable and progressive disease which will eventually lead to death. Gauge the patient's reaction. Discuss palliative care in the context of how it can help the patient achieve his/her goals. Stress the positive aspects of palliative care – living as well as possible for as long as possible.

## GP Notes:

**Basic rules of symptom control:** Symptom control must be tailored to the needs of the individual.
* Carefully diagnose the cause of the symptom
* Explain the symptom to the patient
* Discuss treatment options
* Set realistic goals
* Anticipate likely problems
* Review regularly

⚠ Death is the natural end to life – not a failure of medicine.

## Advice for patients: Information and support

**Macmillan Cancer Support** ☎ 0808 808 0000
🖥 www.macmillan.org.uk

## GMS Contract

| Records 13 | There is a system to alert the out-of-hours service or duty doctor to patients dying at home | 2 points |
|---|---|---|

# Ethics and palliative care

'Ethics' is the critical reflection on morality. Ethical principles are not laws, but guiding principles, which should direct doctors and other health care professionals in their work and decision making. The ethics of end of life decisions is a complex field worthy of a volume of its own – this page aims to address just the common issues likely to affect GPs on a day-to-day basis.

**Communication and disclosure:** Patients have a right to an honest and full explanation of their situation and should be told as much or as little as they want to know – they also have a right to decline information.

Communication should always be with the patient direct unless:
- An interpreter is needed – where possible use professional interpreters who will translate directly and not embellish information with their own opinions – always look the patient not the interpreter in the eye.
- The patient is not competent.
- The patient has delegated the responsibility to a family member.

**Withholding/withdrawing treatment:** The goal of palliative care is to maintain quality of life while neither hastening nor postponing death. Whether it is appropriate to offer or withhold/withdraw a particular treatment depends on what is in the patient's best interests i.e. the balance between possible benefits and potential risks. It is often a difficult and complex decision based on individual clinical circumstances.

🛈 Futile therapy with no chance of benefit is never justified. Withholding or withdrawal of futile therapy from the terminally ill is not active euthanasia (📖 p.234) – the intention is to allow death to occur naturally, not to deliberately terminate life.

**'Double effects':** Medications given for the relief of distressing pain or symptoms may, on occasions, hasten the moment of death, the 'double effect'. However, there is no evidence that good palliative medicine shortens life and effective symptom control is just as likely to extend as shorten life. Providing that appropriate drugs are given for appropriate medical reasons and in appropriate doses, this is not euthanasia – the hastening of death may or may not be foreseen, but is never intended.

## Examples:

**Antibiotics for chest infection:** Whether to prescribe antibiotics for chest infection in patients who are terminally ill depends on many factors, including nearness to death and wishes of the patient and family. If the antibiotics will merely prolong the dying process, they are probably best withheld. If they will control distressing symptoms unresponsive to other measures (e.g. pyrexia, delirium) they may be of benefit.

**Fluids for dehydration:** Whether to supplement fluids for patients who cannot drink adequate amounts depends on clinical state and wishes of the patient and/or family.

Dehydration in patients who are unable to take fluids but are not in the final stages of their disease causes thirst, dry mouth, and postural hypotension. In these patients, parenteral hydration is always warranted.

For dying patients it is a much more difficult decision and the 'right' answer will depend on individual circumstances. There is often an overwhelming need for relatives and staff to give a dying patient food and water but do not allow this to override the patient's need for comfort.

• Dry mouth can be palliated topically and dying patients do not tend to complain of thirst.
• Avoiding overhydration in dying patients may improve comfort as it decreases urine output, pulmonary secretions, GI secretions, oedema, and effusions.
• Giving fluids might worsen the situation and prolong the dying process.
• Drips can give false hope to the patient and/or family, and act as a physical barrier between patient and family.

Explain the advantages and disvantages of artificial hydration. Seek the opinions of the patient (if practicable) and/or relatives. If a decision is made to artificially hydrate, consider subcutaneous fluids.

**Euthanasia and physician-assisted suicide:** 📖 p.234.

**Further information:**

**Beauchamp and Childress** *Principles of Biomedical Ethics* (5th edition-2001). Oxford University Press ISBN: 0195143329

| Table 4.1 The four principles of medical ethics | |
|---|---|
| **Beneficence** | **Autonomy** |
| Whatever is done or said is for the patient's good | Respect for the person and his/her rights to self-determination |
| *e.g. benefits of treatment must outweigh risks* | *e.g. it is the patient's right to decide which treatments they do or do not have* |
| **Non-maleficence** | **Justice** |
| Whatever is done or said will do the patient no harm | Equitable allocation of healthcare resources according to need – not wealth, class, creed, or colour |
| *e.g. never lie to patients* | |

# Breaking bad news

It is never easy to break bad news but, sadly, GPs have to do it frequently.

## Why is breaking bad news hard?

- *Admission of failure:* When we tell patients bad news it is often an admission that we have failed. When we fail we naturally question what we have done and when looking at our practice in retrospect it is easy to find fault. Feelings of guilt are common.
- *Fear of the reaction of the patient:* We all have a desire to avoid unpleasantness but sharing information with patients may be a positive way forwards. Even if news is bad it gives the patient control of the situation.

| Guidelines for sharing bad news with a patient | |
| --- | --- |
| **DO:** | **DON'T:** |
| <ul><li>Plan the consultation as far as possible. Check the facts first and ensure you have all the information. Ensure privacy and freedom from interruption.</li><li>Set aside enough time.</li><li>Ask if the patient would like a relative or friend with them. Make sure you introduce yourself and find out their name and relationship to the patient.</li><li>Make eye contact – watch for non-verbal messages. Sit at the same level as the patient.</li><li>Use simple and straightforward language.</li><li>Allow silence, tears, or anger.</li><li>Be prepared to go over facts again.</li><li>Answer questions.</li><li>Reflect on what the patient or relative have said to allow you to modify your understanding of their feelings.</li><li>Take into account the patients current health e.g. if in pain, then sort out the pain and schedule a further discussion when the patient is more comfortable.</li><li>Offer ongoing support.</li></ul> | <ul><li>Lie or 'fudge' the issue.</li><li>Get your facts wrong.</li><li>Break bad news in public.</li><li>Give the impression of being rushed or distant.</li><li>Give too much information. It is better to be concise – the finer points can be filled in later.</li><li>Interrupt or argue.</li><li>Say that 'nothing can be done' – there is always something that can be done.</li><li>Meet anger with anger.</li><li>Say you know how they feel – you don't.</li><li>Be frightened to admit you don't know something.</li><li>Use medical jargon.</li><li>Leave the patient with no follow on contact.</li><li>Agree to withhold information from the patient.</li></ul> |

**GP Notes: Frequently asked questions about breaking bad news**

### What if the relatives do not want you to tell the patient?

- With adults of sound mind, information is confidential to the patient and can only be released, even to close relatives, with the patients permission.
- Relatives who say they don't want the patient to know often do so to protect their relative. It is important to recognize they know your patient best.
- First, explore their worries and point out the difficulties of the patient not knowing.
- Often once a relative realizes that the patient knows things are not right and needs help and support to face the situation, they come round to the patient being told.
- Stress that you will not lie to a patient if asked a direct question.

### How do you know if the patient wants to know?

Most people (80–90%) *do* want to know. Assume this is the case and then feel your way carefully. Give the patient ample opportunity to say they don't want to know.

### How do you respond to questions you can't answer?

The best way to deal with this is to say you don't have all the answers but will answer when you can. Find out what you can and say when you don't know.

# Bereavement, grief, and coping with loss

### Models of grief:
**Traditional model:** Four phases to 'recovery':
- *Initial shock:* sense of unreality, detachment, disbelief, or 'numbness'. Lasts from hours to days.
- *Yearning:* pangs of grief, episodes of intense pining and a desire to search interspersed with anxiety, guilt, and self-reproach.
- *Despair:* The permanence of the loss is realised. Despair and apathy, social withdrawal, poor concentration, pessimism about the future.
- *Recovery:* rebuilding of an identity and purpose in life.

**Recent models:** Grief is an oscillation between loss- and restoration-focused behaviour, demonstrated by swings in mood, thoughts and behaviour between memories of the dead person and 'getting on with life'. Avoidance or denial of loss is common and part of the process.

### Health consequences of bereavement:
- ↑ *mortality* (CHD cirrhosis, suicide, accidents) – particularly in first 6mo. *Risk factors:* ♂>♀, age <65y., lower social class.
- *Mental health problems:* depression, anxiety, ↑ risk of suicide, substance abuse, identification reaction (hyperchondriacal disorder – symptoms mimic those of deceased e.g. chest pain if died from MI), insomnia, self-neglect.
- *Physical problems:* fatigue, aches and pains (e.g. headaches, musculoskeletal pain), appetite change, GI symptoms, ↓ immune response (↑ minor infection).
- *Others:* interference with family life, education and employment, social isolation/loneliness, ↓ income.

**Bereaved children:** Children understand what death is by 8y. and even children of 2–3y. have some understanding of death. Exclusion makes children isolated and often makes the death of someone they have known more, not less, painful. Prepare children for a death if possible and give them a chance to have their questions answered. If a child has problems, seek specialist help.

**Abnormal grief reactions:** Whether a grief reaction is normal or abnormal depends on individual circumstances – including personality, situation surrounding death, and cultural expectations. Recognized patterns of abnormal grief are:
- Inhibited grief – grief is absent or minimal
- Delayed grief – late onset
- Prolonged or chronic grief – inability to rebuild life in any way

### If abnormal grief is suspected:
- Monitor carefully
- Consider referral for bereavement counselling e.g. to CRUSE
- Consider clinical depression or post-traumatic stress disorder
- If symptoms are persistent or worsening despite treatment, or if there is suicidal risk, refer to psychiatry for specialist advice

### Role of the Primary Care Team:
- Develop a practice policy for dealing with bereaved patients.
- Flag notes.
- Consider staff training and employing active follow up of bereaved patients.
- If the person who has died is registered with the practice, ensure all medical referrals/appointments are cancelled.

### Risk factors for poor outcome after bereavement:
**Predisposing factors:**
- Multiple prior bereavements
- History of mental illness (e.g. depression, anxiety, suicidal attempts or threats)
- Ambivalent or dependent relationship with the deceased
- Low self-esteem
- Being male
- Poor social or family support

### Situations where the circumstances of death may cause particular problems for the bereaved:
- Sudden or unexpected death
- Death of parent when child or adolescent
- Multiple deaths (e.g. disasters)
- Miscarriage, death of baby, child or sibling
- Cohabiting partners, same sex partners, extramarital relationship
- Death due to AIDS or suicide
- Deaths where those bereaved may be responsible
- Deaths from murder, with high media profile or involving legal proceedings
- Where a postmortem and/or inquest is required

93

**Advice for patients: Useful contacts**

**CRUSE** ☎ 0844 477 9400 (young people: 0808 808 1677)
🖳 www.crusebereavementcare.org.uk
**Royal College of Psychiatrists** information leaflet. Available at
🖳 www.rcpsych.ac.uk
**National Association of Widows** ☎ 024 7663 4848
🖳 www.widows.uk.net

# Chapter 5

# Symptom control and clinical scenarios in palliative care

# A–Z index of palliative care symptoms/scenarios

| Symptom | Page reference |
|---------|----------------|
| **G/H** | |
| Gastro-intestinal bleeding | 📖 p.118 |
| Haematemesis | GI bleeding – 📖 p.118 |
| Haematuria | 📖 p.132 |
| Haemoptysis | 📖 p.140 |
| Haemorrhage | Massive bleeding – 📖 p.98 |
| Hiccup | Mouth problems – 📖 p.108 |
| Hypercalcaemia | 📖 p.144 |
| **I/J/K/L** | |
| ICP (raised) | Neurological and orthopaedic problems – 📖 p.148 |
| Impotence | Sexual health – 📖 p.136 |
| Incontinence | 📖 p.128 |
| Insomnia | 📖 p.160 |
| Itch | 📖 p.105 |
| Liver capsule pain | 📖 p.101 |
| Lymphoedema | 📖 p.156 |
| **M/N** | |
| Mouth problems | 📖 p.108 |
| Myoclonic twitching | Neurological and orthopaedic problems – 📖 p.149 |
| Nausea and vomiting | 📖 p.114 |
| Nerve pain | 📖 p.40 and 101 |
| Noisy breathing | Death rattle – 📖 p.192 |
| **O/P/Q/R** | |
| Obstruction (bowel) | Other GI problems – 📖 p.122 |
| Pressure area care | Wound care – 📖 p.158 |
| Pulmonary embolus | Venous thromboembolism – 📖 p.152 |
| Reduced libido | Sexual health – 📖 p.134 |
| Retention | Overflow – 📖 p.130 |
| **S/T** | |
| Sexual health | 📖 p.134 |
| Sore mouth | Mouth problems – 📖 p.108 |
| Spinal cord compression | Neurological and orthopaedic problems – 📖 p.149 |
| Stoma care | Patients with ostomies – 📖 p.126 |
| Stridor | 📖 p.138 |
| Superior vena cava obstruction | Breathlessness – 📖 p.143 |
| Sweating | General debility – 📖 p.104 |
| Syringe drivers | 📖 p.36 and 194–7 |
| Tenesmus | Other GI problems – 📖 p.124 |
| Terminal phase | The last 48h. – 📖 p.188 |
| Terminal restlessness | The last 48h. – 📖 p.190 |
| **U/V/W** | |
| Vaginal soreness | Sexual health – 📖 p.134 |
| Vomiting | Nausea and vomiting – 📖 p.114 |
| Weakness | General debility – 📖 p.104 |
| Wound care | 📖 p.158 |

# Emergencies

Some acute events in advanced disease must be treated as an emergency. While unnecessary hospital admission may cause distress for patients/ carers, missed emergency treatment of reversible conditions can be disastrous.

## Questions to ask when managing emergencies:

- What is the problem?
- Can it be reversed?
- What effect will reversal have on the patient's overall condition?
- Could active treatment maintain/improve this patient's quality of life?
- What do you think is the 'right' thing to do?
- What does the patient want?
- What do the carers want?

| Table 5.1 Emergencies in advanced disease | |
|---|---|
| **Condition** | **Emergency management** |
| Hypercalcaemia ☐ p.144 | Depending on the general state of the patient, make a decision whether to treat the hypercalcaemia or not. *If a decision is made not to treat:* provide symptom control and do not check the serum calcium again. *Active treatment:* depends on level of symptoms and calcium: <br> • Asymptomatic patient with corrected calcium <3mmol/l – monitor. <br> • Symptomatic and/or corrected calcium > 3mmol/l – arrange treatment with IV fluids/bisphosphonates via oncologist/palliative care team as an emergency. |
| Bone fracture | Give analgesia. Unless in a terminal state, confirm the fracture on X-ray and refer to orthopaedics or radiotherapy urgently for consideration of fixation (long bones, wrist, neck of femur) and/or radiotherapy (rib fractures, vertebral fractures). |
| Massive bleeding <br> Haematuria – ☐ p.132 <br> Haemoptysis – ☐ p.140 <br> GI bleeding – ☐ p.118 <br> Wounds – ☐ p.159 | Make a decision whether the cause of the bleed is treatable or a terminal event. *Active treatment:* Call for emergency ambulance support. Lie flat. Gain IV access and give IV fluids if available. *No active treatment:* Stay with the patient, give sedative medication (e.g. midazolam 10–40mg s/cut or IM or diazepam 10–20mg pr). Support the carers. Consider diamorphine 2–10mg s/cut if the patient is in pain. |
| Acute breathlessness ☐ p.142 | Consider reversible causes: anaemia, pneumonia, pleural effusion, exacerbation of COPD, heart failure, PE, superior vena cava obstruction. *Palliative measures:* morphine 2.5–5mg prn (or ↑ background opioid dose by 30–50%) or consider diamorphine/morphine syringe driver with midazolam 5–10mg over 24h. |

**Table 5.1** (*Contd.*)

| Condition | Emergency management |
|---|---|
| *Spinal cord compression* 📖 p.149 | Presents with back pain worse on movement and neurological symptoms e.g. constipation, weak legs, incontinence of urine.<br><br>Prompt treatment (<24–48h. from 1st neurological symptoms) is needed if there is any hope of restoring function. Treat with oral dexamethasone 16mg/d. and refer urgently for radiotherapy unless in final stages of disease. |
| *Pain* 📖 p.100–101 | Breakthrough of pre-existing opioid-responsive pain: give a stat dose of opioid = 1/6th total opioid dose in the last 24h. Acts in <30min. Repeat if ineffective. Reassess cause of pain and consider alternative analgesic approaches. |
| *Opiate overdose* 📖 p.35 | *If respiratory rate ≥ 8/min. and patient is easily rousable and not cyanosed* – review if condition worsens. Consider reducing or omitting the next regular dose of opioid.<br><br>*If respiratory rate < 8/min., and/or the patient is barely rousable/unconscious and/or cyanosed*, dilute a standard ampoule containing naloxone 400mcgm to 10ml with sodium chloride 0.9%. Administer 2ml (80mcg) IV every 2min. until respiratory status is satisfactory to a maximum of 10mg naloxone. If respiratory function still doesn't improve, question diagnosis.<br><br>❶ Further boluses may be necessary once respiratory function improves as naloxone is shorter acting than morphine. |
| *Fitting* | Ensure the airway is clear and turn the patient into the recovery position. Prevent onlookers from restraining the fitting patient.<br><br>Treat fitting with diazepam 5–10mg IV or pr.<br><br>If >1 seizure without the patient regaining consciousness or fitting continues >20min. repeat diazepam every 15min. until fitting is controlled. Unless in a very terminal condition, admit.<br><br>Support carers.<br><br>Consider checking BM. Depending on clinical state, consider referral for further investigation if first fit. |
| *Terminal restlessness/ agitation* 📖 p.190 | *Causes:* Pain/discomfort, myoclonic jerks 2° to opioid toxicity, biochemical causes (e.g. ↑ $Ca^{2+}$, uraemia), psychological/spiritual distress, full bladder or rectum.<br><br>*Management:*<br>• Treat reversible causes e.g. catheterization for retention, hyoscine to dry up secretions.<br><br>• If still restless, treat with a sedative. This does NOT shorten life but makes the patient and any relatives in attendance more comfortable.<br><br>*Suitable drugs:* haloperidol 1–3mg tds po; diazepam 2–10mg tds po, midazolam (10–100mg/24h. via syringe driver or 5mg stat) or levomepromazine (12.5–50mg/24h. via syringe driver or 6.25mg stat). |

# Pain control

Pain control is the cornerstone of palliative care. Cancer pain is multifactorial – be aware of physical and psychological factors.

**Principles of pain control:** 📖 pp.12–19

**Pain-relieving drugs:** 📖 pp.20–45

**Summary of management of specific types of pain:** Table 5.2

**Back pain and spinal cord compression:** Spinal cord compression occurs in 5% of patients with cancer (📖 p.149). 90% present with back pain – often preceding any neurological symptoms. Prompt treatment is needed if there is any hope of restoring function.

## Presentation:
- Often back pain, worse on movement, appears before neurology.
- Neurological symptoms/signs can be non-specific – constipation, weak legs, urinary hesitancy.
- Lesions above L1 (lower end of spinal cord) may produce UMN signs (e.g. ↑ tone and reflexes) and a sensory level.
- Lesions below L1 may produce LMN signs (↓ tone & reflexes) and perianal numbness (cauda equina syndrome).

## Management: Ask:
1. *Is there a reasonable likelihood of spinal cord compression?* Maintain a *high* level of suspicion in all cancer patients who complain of back pain – especially those with known bony metastases or tumours likely to metastasize to bone (e.g. myeloma, and cancers of the prostate, breast and bronchus).
2. *Would this patient benefit from emergency investigation and treatment?* Treat with oral dexamethasone 16mg/d. and refer as an emergency for surgery/radiotherapy unless in final stages of disease.

**Bladder pain:** Discomfort in the suprapubic area ± dysuria, frequency, nocturia, urgency and/or urine retention/incontinence.

## Causes of bladder pain:
- *UTI* – bacterial (including TB if immunocompromized), fungal.
- *Tumour* – bladder, urethra, pelvic mass 2° to other tumour e.g. bowel, ovary.
- *Treatment related* e.g. 2° to radiotherapy, chemotherapy or immunotherapy, 2° to a blocked or infected catheter.
- *Calculus* – bladder stones.
- *Bladder irritability/spasm* – may be idiopathic or due to contraction around the balloon of an indwelling catheter, blood clots, tumour, or infection.
- *Retention of urine* – check bladder is not enlarged

In addition, dysuria and/or ↑ frequency may be caused by genital herpes, urethritis, and/or vaginitis.

**Management:** Where possible treat the cause. In all cases, ↑ fluids and encourage regular toileting. Drug options – Table 5.2.

## Table 5.2 Management of specific types of pain

| Type of pain | Management |
|---|---|
| Bone pain | • Try NSAIDs and/or strong opioids<br>• Consider referral for palliative radiotherapy, strontium treatment (prostate cancer) or IV bisphosphonates (↓ pain in myeloma, breast and prostate cancer)<br>• Refer to orthopaedics if any lytic metastases at risk of fracture, for consideration of pinning |
| Abdominal pain | • Constipation is the commonest cause – 📖 p.120<br>• Colic – try loperamide 2–4mg qds po, hyoscine hydrobromide 300mcgm tds s/ling, or Hyoscine butylbromide (Buscopan®) 20–60mg/24h. via syringe driver.<br>• Liver capsule pain – use dexamethasone 4–8mg/d. Titrate dose ↓ to the minimum that controls pain. Alternatively try an NSAID + PPI cover.<br>• Gastric distention – may be helped by an antacid ± an antifoaming agent (e.g. Asilone®). Alternatively a prokinetic may help e.g. metoclopramide or domperidone 10mg tds before meals.<br>• Upper GI tumour – often neuropathic element of pain—if not controlled – refer to palliative care team<br>• Consider drug causes– NSAIDs are a common iatrogenic cause<br>• Acute/subacute obstruction – 📖 p.122 |
| Neuropathic pain | • Often burning/shooting and may not respond to simple analgesia.<br>• Titrate to the maximum tolerated dose of opioid e.g. tramadol, oxycodone<br>• If inadequate, add a nerve pain killer e.g. amitriptyline 10–25mg nocte increasing as needed every 2wk. to 75–150mg. Alternatives include carbamazepine, gabapentin, pregabalin, phenytoin, sodium valproate and clonazepam<br>• If pain is due to nerve compression due to tumour, dexamethasone 4–8mg od may help.<br>• Other options: TENS; acupuncture; nerve block |
| Rectal pain | • Topical drugs e.g. rectal steroids<br>• Tricyclic antidepressants e.g. amitriptyline 10–100mg nocte<br>• Anal spasms – glyceryl trinitrate ointment 0.1–0.2% bd<br>• Referral for local radiotherapy |
| Muscle pain | • Paracetamol and/or NSAIDs<br>• Muscle relaxants e.g. diazepam 5–10mg od, baclofen 5–10mg tds, dantrolene 25mg od increasing at weekly intervals to 75mg tds<br>• Physiotherapy, aromatherapy, relaxation, heat pads |
| Bladder pain/spasm | • Treat reversible causes. ↑ fluids. Toilet regularly<br>• Try tolterodine 2mg bd, propiverine 15mg od/bd/tds, or trospium 20mg bd<br>• Amitriptyline 10–75mg nocte is often effective<br>• If catheterized – try instilling 20ml of intravesical bupivacaine 0.25% for 15min. tds or oxybutynin 5ml in 30ml od/bd/tds<br>• NSAIDs can also be useful<br>• Steroids e.g. dexamethasone 4–8mg od may ↓ tumour-related bladder inflammation<br>• In the terminal situation, hyoscine butylbromide 60–120mg/24h. or glycopyrronium 0.4–0.8mg/24h. s/cut can be helpful (higher doses can be given under specialist supervision) |
| Pain of short duration | • e.g. dressing changes – try a short-acting opioid e.g. fentanyl citrate 200mcgm lozenge sucked for 15min prior to the procedure or a breakthrough dose of oral morphine 20min. prior to the procedure. |

# Use of steroids

GPs are often reluctant to use steroids in palliative care situations, partly due to unfamiliarity with their use, and partly due to worries about initiation and monitoring within a primary care situation.

**Use and administration:** Table 5.3
- Give initially for a 1wk. trial and stop if not effective.
- Often started at high dose to suppress disease process and stepped down with improvement.
- Use the minimum dose that controls symptoms for maintenance.
- Where possible, prescribe oral steroids as a single dose in the morning (after breakfast) to ↓ circadian rhythm disturbance.
- Dexamethasone is the corticosteroid of choice in advanced disease because of its reduced tablet burden on patients.
- Prednisolone is most commonly used to treat chronic disease e.g. asthma, inflammatory bowel disease or rheumatoid arthritis.
- Supply with a 'steroid card'.
- In the terminal care situation, inability to swallow oral medication is often the factor which leads to stopping steroids. Consider use of soluble preparations. Weigh up the burden of continuing against the risks – continue s/cut steroids only if there is a clear ongoing benefit.

**Side effects:** Doses of dexamethasone >4mg od are likely to result in significant side effects after a few weeks. Doses ≤4mg od are usually well tolerated in patients with a prognosis of months.
- ↑BP
- Osteoporosis ± fracture – long-term use or recurrent short courses
- Proximal muscle wasting (worse with dexamethasone than prednisolone – consider switching if a problem)
- Euphoria
- Paranoid states or depression – especially if previous psychiatric disorder
- Peptic ulceration – ↑ risk if also taking NSAIDs. Soluble or enteric coated (EC) versions may ↓ risk. Consider protecting gastric mucosa with a PPI – especially if taking a NSAID concurrently
- Suppression of clinical signs—may allow diseases e.g. septicaemia to reach advanced stage before being recognized
- Spread of infection e.g. chickenpox, oral thrush
- Hyperglycaemia in non-diabetic patients (consider weekly urine monitoring for glucose followed up by fasting blood glucose if positive) and worsening of diabetic control in diabetic patients
- Cushing's syndrome – moon face, striae, and acne
- Adrenal atrophy – can persist for years after stopping long-term steroids – illness or surgical emergencies may require steroid supplements
- Frail skin, which bruises easily
- $Na^+$ and water retention; $K^+$ loss

> 🛈 If patients are expected to be on oral steroids for >3mo. (e.g. cerebral tumour where prognosis is uncertain, or chronic inflammatory disease e.g. rheumatoid arthritis), consider osteoporosis prophylaxis with an oral bisphosphonate.

| Table 5.3 Use of steroids in palliative care | |
|---|---|
| **Indication for use** | **Daily dose of dexamethasone** |
| Anorexia<br>Weakness<br>Pain (where caused by tumoural oedema)<br>Improvement in well-being/mood | 2–4mg |
| Nerve compression pain<br>Liver capsule pain<br>Nausea<br>Bowel obstruction<br>Post-radiation inflammation | 4–8mg |
| ↑ Intracranial pressure<br>Superior vena cava obstruction<br>Carcinomatosa lymphangitis<br>Spinal cord compression | 12–16mg |
| ↑ dose for patients on liver-enzyme-inducing drugs e.g. phenytoin, carbamazepine or phenobarbital | |

**Withdrawal of steroids:** Stop abruptly if the patient has received treatment for ≤3wk. and is not included in the patient groups described below.

*Withdraw gradually if the patient has:*
- Recently had repeated steroid courses (particularly if taken for >3wk.)
- Taken a short course <1y. after stopping long-term therapy
- Other possible causes of adrenal suppression
- Received >4mg dexamethasone or >40mg prednisolone per day
- Been given repeat doses in the evening
- Received treatment with steroids for >3wk.

During corticosteroid withdrawal, ↓ dose rapidly to physiological levels (~ prednisolone 7.5mg od or 4mg dexamethasone od) – thereafter ↓ more slowly. Assess during withdrawal to ensure symptoms don't recur (or treat symptoms if steroid withdrawal in the terminal days of disease).

103

**GP Notes: Steroid cards**

Should be carried at all times by patients on oral or high doses of inhaled steroids. The card:
- Informs other practitioners your patient is on steroids *and*
- Gives the patient advice on use of steroids and risk of infection

*Obtaining steroid cards:*
- England and Wales: Department of Health ☎ 08701 555 455
- Scotland: Banner Business Supplies ☎ 01506 448 440

# General debility

**Weakness, fatigue and drowsiness:** *Asthenia* is characterized by fatigue or easy tiring and ↓ sustainability of performance, generalized weakness resulting in ↓ ability to initiate movement, and mental fatigue with poor concentration, impaired memory and emotional lability. It is almost a universal symptom.

**Reversible causes:**
- Drugs – opioids, benzodiazepines, steroids (proximal muscle weakness), diuretics (dehydration and biochemical abnormalities), antihypertensives (postural hypotension)
- Emotional problems – depression, anxiety, fear, apathy
- Hypercalcaemia
- Other biochemical abnormalities – DM, electrolyte disturbance, uraemia, liver disease, thyroid dysfunction
- Anaemia (📖 p.106)
- Poor nutrition
- Infection
- Prolonged bed rest
- Raised intracranial pressure (drowsiness only)

**Management:**
- Treat reversible causes.
- Encourage ↑ gentle exercise
- If drowsiness and fatigue persist consider a trial of dexamethasone 4–6mg/d. or an antidepressant. Although steroids make muscle wasting worse, they may improve general fatigue and improve mobility.
- Psychological support of patients and carers – empathy, explanation.
- Physical support – referral to physiotherapist, review of aids and appliances, review of home layout (possibly with referral to OT), review of home care arrangements.
- Advice on modification of lifestyle.

**Fever and sweating:** Sweats and fevers can occur alone or together. As well as interrupting sleep, they are very uncomfortable.

**Causes:** Box 5.1

**Management:** Direct treatment at the cause, wherever possible.
- Nursing care – regular sponging, washing, fanning, encourage oral fluids.
- Paracetamol 1g qds prn – may not be effective for neoplastic fevers.
- Alternatives include:
  - NSAIDs e.g. ibuprofen 400mg tds.
  - Ondansetron 8mg bd.
  - Aspirin 300–600mg qds.
  - Antimuscarinics e.g. oxybutynin.
  - SSRIs e.g. fluoxetine 20mg od (for sweats).
  - SNRIs e.g. venlafaxine SR 75mg od (for hormone related sweats).
  - Megestrol 20mg od/bd (for hot flushes).
  - Thalidomide 100–200mg nocte – for neoplastic fever (capsules must not be handled directly by women of child-bearing age – specialist prescription only).
  - High-dose steroids – sweating in chronic lymphatic leukaemia.
  - Cimetidine 200–800mg nocte – sweating related to opioid use.

**Itch:** Itching is a common and uncomfortable problem for many terminally ill patients. Causes include:
- Skin disease—e.g. eczema, psoriasis, flea bites, scabies
- Allergy—e.g. urticaria, contact dermatitis
- Haematological disease—iron deficiency, lymphoma, polycythaemia
- Liver disease—biliary obstruction
- Chronic renal failure
- Thyroid disease—usually hypothyroidism.

**Management:** Try to find the cause and treat where possible.

*General measures:*
- Keep skin well moisturized—use bath/shower emollients, apply moisturizers frequently (e.g. aqueous cream) use as soap substitutes, avoid detergents and soaps.
- Avoid exacerbating factors e.g. keep bath water cool, wear cotton, avoid prickly clothing, clip nails short.
- Try soothing preparations e.g. adding bicarbonate of soda to the bath, calamine lotion, moisturizers with anti-itch agents in them.

*Drug measures:* Consider:
- Antihistamines—sedating antihistamines (e.g. chlorphenamine 4mg tds) tend to be more effective than non-sedating ones
- Sedatives e.g. diazepam 2mg tds or chlorpromazine 10–25mg tds/qds
- Cimetidine 400mg bd (especially for lymphoma)
- Paroxetine 20mg od for paraneoplastic or morphine itch.

**Obstructive jaundice:** Consider referral for stent. Otherwise cholestyramine 6–8g/d., aluminium hydroxide mixture 10–15ml tds/qds or ondansetron 8mg od may be helpful.

🕐 If simple measures aren't succeeding, refer to palliative care or dermatology for advice.

---

### Box 5.1 Causes of fever and/or sweats

| Non-malignant causes: | Neoplastic fever: |
| --- | --- |
| • Systemic infection (e.g. chest infection, UTI) | • Common (up to 60% of patients with malignancy) |
| • Menopausal symptoms | • Particularly common with lymphoma, leukaemia, hypernephroma and tumours with liver metastases |
| • Thyroid disease | |
| • Connective tissue and autoimmune disease e.g. RA, SLE | |
| • Drugs (e.g. opioids, chemotherapy agents, tamoxifen, calcium channel blockers, antibiotics) | |
| • DVT/PE | |
| • Blood transfusion | |
| • Hypoglycaemia | |
| • Shock e.g. due to MI, bleeding | |

# Anorexia and cachexia

Anorexia is the absence or loss of appetite for food. Cachexia is a condition of profound weight loss and catabolic loss of muscle and adipose tissue – usually compounded by a chronic ↓ nutritional intake. Anorexia and/or cachexia occurs in ~ 70% of patients with advanced cancer.

## Primary causes:

Anorexia cachexia syndrome is a multifactorial syndrome caused by disease and autoimmune responses to chronic illness. It is often characterized by muscle loss and a raised CRP and lowered albumin. Treatment options are limited though trials are currently underway.

## Reversible secondary causes:

- Dysphagia e.g. oral thrush, sore/dry mouth, upper GI mass (may be treated with a bypass procedure, radiotherapy and/or chemotherapy)
- Nausea or vomiting
- Constipation
- Pain
- Anxiety or depression
- Physical inability to prepare or eat meals (e.g. unable to cook, poor fitting teeth)

## Management:

- Treat reversible causes where possible
- ↓ psychological distress and treat depression
- Address physical barriers to eating e.g. meals on wheels
- Consider referral to a dietician for advice on diet
- Advise small, appetising meals frequently in comfortable surroundings

## Drugs that may be helpful:

- Alcohol pre-meals.
- Metoclopramide or domperidone 10mg tds pre-meals – to prevent feeling of satiety caused by gastric stasis.
- Trials of dexamethasone 2–4mg od or prednisolone 15–30mg od – ↑ appetite and well-being in 80% but the effect is usually short-lived. Use the minimum effective dose. If there is no response after 7–10d. stop.
- Progestogens[C] e.g. megesterol acetate 80–160mg od or medroxyprogesterone acetate 400mg od, ↑ appetite in 80%—onset of effect is slower than with corticosteroids but lasts longer. Side effects include oedema, ↑BP and insomnia.

**Nutritional support:** Although nutritional support in the form of nasogastric or IV feeding may improve weight and well-being in the short term, it can only be justified as a short-term measure prior to or after definitive treatment e.g. preparing for/recovering from surgery or awaiting chemotherapy.

**Hydration in the dying patient:** 📖 p.89

**Anaemia:** Don't check for anaemia if there is no intention to treat.
• *If Hb <10g/dl and symptomatic:* treat any reversible cause (e.g. iron deficiency, GI bleeding 2° to NSAIDs). Consider transfusion.
• *If transfused:* Record whether any benefit is derived (as if not further transfusions are futile) and duration of benefit (if <3 wk. – repeat transfusions are impractical). Monitor for return of symptoms, repeat FBC and arrange repeat transfusion as needed.

---

### GP Notes: Food supplements on prescription

In certain conditions, some foods have characteristics of drugs and the Advisory Committee on Borderline Substances (ACBS) advises as to the circumstances in which such substances may be regarded as drugs.

Many food supplements are available for treatment of dysphagia, malabsorption and disease-related malnutrition e.g.
• Abbott – Ensure®, Enrich®, Enlive®, Formance®
• Nutricia clinical – Forticreme®, Fortifresh®, Fortijuce®, Fortimel®, Fortisip®, Polycal®
• Fresenius Kabi – Fresubin®, Calshake®
• SHS – Maxijul®, Duocal®, Duobar®
• Novartis – Resource®, Isosource®, Novasource®
• Nestlé – Clinutren®, Caloreen®

A full list is available in the BNF – Appendix 7 ⌨ www.bnf.org

Endorse prescriptions 'ACBS'.

🔮 In the presence of primary anorexia cachexia syndrome, which is essentially a metabolic problem, these food supplements have little role to play. Unfortunately GPs come under pressure to prescribe food supplements from the point at which cancer is diagonised, even in patients who are eating well. Try to resist prescribing unless you have good reason.

---

### Further information:

**Cochrane** Berenstein and Ortiz Megestrol acetate for the treatment of anorexia-cachexia syndrome 2005.
**European Journal of Palliative Care** Macdonald N Anorexia-cachexia syndrome (2005). **12**(2) Supplement 8–14.

# Mouth problems

Mouth problems affect up to 60% of patients with advanced cancer and can impact greatly on quality of life – both physically and psychologically. The majority of mouth problems seen in palliative care are related to a ↓ in saliva secretion and/or poor oral hygiene.

## Risk factors:
- ↓ oral intake
- Debility and ↓ ability to perform self-care
- Dry mouth (due to medication, radiotherapy, anxiety, mouth breathing, oxygen therapy)
- Dehydration
- Weight loss (results in poor-fitting dentures)
- Anaemia (iron deficiency anaemia causes angular stomatitis and glossitis)
- Vitamin C deficiency (causes gingivitis and bleeding gums)
- Local irradiation
- Chemotherapy
- Local tumour

**Assessment:** Assess regularly for symptoms/signs of mouth problems e.g. altered taste, pain, and/or mouth ulcers, dry mouth, halitosis, thrush or dental problems. Consider checking FBC for iron deficiency anaemia.

## General measures:
- Keep mouth moist – encourage regular sips of fluids and/or rinsing
- Clean teeth/dentures regularly – if the patient is unable to do it for him/herself instruct carers on mouth care
- Gently clean the tongue with a soft toothbrush or sponge
- Apply moisturizing cream or petroleum jelly (Vaseline®) to lips
- Review medication making the mouth sore or dry
- Mouthwashes – saline 0.9% mouthwashes help removal of oral debris and are soothing
- Consider referral to the DN or palliative care home nursing team for advice
- Consider referral to the dentist, ENT or palliative care if symptoms are not settling.

## Specific measures: Table 5.4

**Hiccup:** A distressing symptom. Treatment is often unsatisfactory.
- *General measures:* Rebreathing with a paper bag; pharyngeal stimulation by drinking cold water or taking a teaspoonful of granulated sugar.
- *Peripheral hiccups:* Caused by irritation of the phrenic nerve or diaphragm – try small, frequent meals; metoclopramide (10mg tds); antacids containing dimeticone (e.g. Gaviscon®, Asilone®); dexamethasone (4–12mg/d.); or, ranitidine (150mg bd).
- *Central hiccups:* Due to medullary stimulation e.g. ↑ICP, uraemia – try chlorpromazine (25mg stat then 10–25mg tds/qds), dexamethasone (4–12mg/d.), nifedipine (5–10mg prn or tds) or baclofen (5mg bd/tds). Anticonvulsants e.g. gabapentin may also be effective.

## Table 5.4 Specific measures for treatment of mouth problems

| Problem | Treatment options |
|---------|-------------------|
| Dry mouth | Review medication that might be causing dryness e.g. opioids, antidepressants |
| | Hydrate as well as possible |
| | Consider salivary stimulants (especially pre-meals) – iced water/sucking ice cubes, pineapple chunks, chewing gum, boiled sweets or mints |
| | Consider saliva substitutes e.g. Glandosane® spray, Oralbalance® gel |
| | Radiotherapy induced dryness – consider pilocarpine 5mg po tds (sweating is a common side effect), pilocarpine 4% eye drops in raspberry syrup or peppermint water 2–3 drops po tds (unlicensed) or bethanechol 10mg tds with meals |
| Mouth ulcers/sore patches | Topical analgesia e.g. Teejel®, Bonjela® |
| | Adcortyl in Orabase® paste topically qds after eating and nocte (or orabase paste alone if no aphthous ulceration) |
| | Hydrocortisone lozenges (Corlan®) 1 qds po to ulcerated area |
| | Tetracycline mouthwash – for resistant ulcers— dissolve contents of a 250mg capsule in water and hold in the mouth for 2–3min. bd for 3d. Avoid swallowing. May stain teeth. |
| | Chemotherapy induced ulcers – sucralfate suspension 10ml as mouthwash every 4h. |
| Mouth cancer pain | Try topical NSAIDs e.g. piroxicam melt 20mg od |
| Excessive salivation/drooling | Non-drug treatment – head positioning, suction |
| | Amitriptyline 10–100mg po |
| | Propantheline 15mg tds |
| | β-blockers e.g. atenolol 50mg od |
| | Atropine eye drops 2 drops to mouth qds (unlicensed) |
| Generally sore mouth | Avoid foods that trigger pain e.g. acidic foods |
| | Consider systemic analgesic e.g. NSAID and/or opioids |
| | Difflam® mouthwash 10ml qds (dilute in same amount of water before use if stings) |
| | Soluble aspirin – rinse mouth and swallow – 300–600mg qds if no contraindications |
| | Lidocaine spray, gel or cream – beware of pharyngeal anaesthesia and risk of aspiration |
| | Betadine®, Oraldene® or chlorhexidine 0.2% (Corsodyl®) mouthwash – rinse with 10ml for 1min. bd |
| Oral infection | 📖 p.110 |
| Coated tongue/mouth | Use a soft toothbrush/sponge to clean the tongue |
| | ¼–½ ascorbic acid 1g effervescent tablet/d. can help – place on tongue and allow to dissolve |
| | Fresh pineapple contains enzymes that dissolve the protein coating – try sucking small pieces. |

**Oral thrush (candidiasis):** *Candida albicans* is a virtually uniform commensal of the mouth and GI tract producing opportunistic infection.

**Presentation:** Sore mouth ± loss of taste ± dysphagia. Examination reveals white plaques visible on buccal mucosa which can be wiped off (Figure 5.1) ± angular stomatitis.

*Management:*
- Remove tongue deposits with a toothbrush by brushing 2x/d.
- Treat infection with oral pastilles, suspensions or gels (e.g. nystatin suspension 100,000U/ml 2–5ml qds po, nystatin pastilles 1 qds, miconazole oral gel 25mg/ml qds or amphotericin lozenges 10mg qds – all after food and nocte for 1–2wk.).
- If false teeth, advise to place imidazole gel on the teeth before insertion and sterilize by soaking for >12h. (usually overnight) with dilute hypochlorite solution (e.g. Milton®) to prevent re-infection.
- Reserve systemic treatment for patients with recurrent, extensive, systemic or resistant infection e.g. oral fluconazole 50mg od for 1–2wk.—higher doses or prolonged therapy may be needed if immunosuppressed (seek specialist advice).

**Herpes simplex (HSV) infection:** Transmitted by direct contact with lesions. After initial infection, HSV remains dormant in the nerve ganglia and recurrent eruptions can occur, precipitated by overexposure to sunlight, febrile illnesses, physical or emotional stress, or immunosuppression. The trigger stimulus is often unknown. Diagnosis is usually clinical but can be confirmed with a viral swab of the ulcer if necessary.

*Presentation:*
- Lesions may appear anywhere but are most frequent around the mouth (Figure 5.2), conjunctiva, cornea, and genitalia. They can be very painful—in the mouth, pain may cause dysphagia and dehydration.
- After a prodromal period (generally <6h.) of tingling, discomfort or itching, small tense vesicles appear on an erythematous base. Single clusters vary in size from 0.5–1.5cm, but groups may coalesce.
- Vesicles persist for a few days, then dry, forming a thin yellowish crust. Healing occurs 8–12d. after onset.
- Infection may be accompanied by systemic symptoms e.g. fever, malaise and tender lymph nodes.
- Immunocompromized patients can develop generalized infection with oesophagitis, colitis, perianal ulcers, pneumonia ± neurological signs.

*Management:*
- *Severe infections:* e.g. immunocompromised patients – admit for systemic treatment with aciclovir.
- *Eye involvement:* Refer for urgent ophthalmology assessment. Treatment is with topical ± oral aciclovir.
- *Suppression of recurrent eruptions:* Oral aciclovir (and similar drugs).
- *Cold sores:* Topical aciclovir – if started early. Available OTC.
- *2° infections:* Topical or systemic antibiotics.
- *Pain:* Strong analgesia. Consider opioids if very painful – may need to be given via syringe driver if unable to swallow.
- *Dehydration:* Consider admitting for iv fluids until pain has settled.

## Figure 5.1 Candidiasis of the tongue

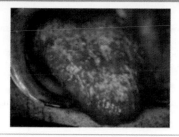

## Figure 5.2 Herpes simplex infection of the lower lip

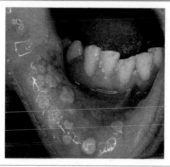

# Dysphagia

Difficulty swallowing food or liquids. Can cause considerable distress to patients and their families.

**Causes:** Box 5.2

**Management:** Treat the cause if possible.

## Post-radiation oesophagitis:
- Avoid smoking, alcohol and spicy food
- Treat any Candida infection (📖 p.110)
- Try an alginate-containing antacid e.g. Gaviscon® or sucralfate suspension
- Try soluble aspirin or soluble paracetamol for pain. If not sufficient, try a NSAID po, buccally or pr (e.g. Piroxicam Melt 20mg od, diclofenac 75mg pr). If pain is severe, consider opioids via syringe driver until pain has settled.
- Oesophageal spasm – try nifedipine 10mg tds.

**Dysphagia due to physical obstruction by tumour bulk:** Consider urgent referral back to oncology or surgery.
- Stenting may help e.g. Celestin tube for oesophageal cancer.
- Chemotherapy/radiotherapy may decrease tumour bulk and give temporary relief.

## Dysphagia due to functional obstruction from neurological deficit:
- Ask speech therapy to assess – Is there a risk of aspiration? Are there any specific techniques to aid safe swallowing?
- If the patient is hungry and wishes to be fed, consider referral for a percutaneous endoscopic gastrostomy (PEG) – see below.
- If the patient does not wish to have a PEG, ask whether s/he would like subcutaneous fluids and treat symptomatically with mouth care, anxiolytics, analgesia, and sedation as needed.

## Gastrostomies:
- Feeding gastrostomies are sometimes used prior to aggressive treatment to improve functional status and the ability to tolerate treatment for malignancies of the head and neck or oesophagus.
- Gastrostomies can be used to improve nutrition and quality of life e.g in patients with MND – especially if death is not imminent – but should only be inserted after careful multidisciplinary discussion involving the patient and their family.
- Ethical dilemmas can arise towards the end of life when gastrostomy feeding may prolong an uncomfortable dying period. Reducing or stopping artificial feeding may then need to be discussed (📖 p.88).
- There is no evidence that routine insertion of feeding tubes in the dying either extends life or improves symptoms, but it can be demanded by families.

🔴 For patients with impaired lung function, PEG insertion carries high mortality. Radiographically inserted gastrostomy (RIG) is an alternative to PEG and avoids endoscopy or sedation.

### Box 5.2 Causes of dysphagia

**Acute:**
- Acute throat infection (e.g. pharyngitis, glandular fever, tonsillitis) ± quinsy
- Epiglottitis
- Foreign body in throat
- Post-radiation oesophagitis

**Progressive:**
- *Within the oesophagus:*
  - Oesophageal/stomach cancer
  - Chronic benign stricture
  - Achalasia
  - Pharyngeal pouch
  - Plummer–Vinson syndrome
  - Oesophageal perforation.
- *Compression from outside:*
  - Enlarged mediastinal LNs
  - Lung cancer
  - Enlarged left atrium
  - Large retrosternal goitre
  - Thoracic aneurysm.
- *Other:*
  - Bulbar palsy
  - Myasthenia gravis
  - Hysteria/anxiety state.

### Advice for patients: Looking after an oesophageal stent to prevent it blocking

- Don't rush eating.
- Have soft food in small mouthfuls and chew it well.
- Drink a little during and after meals – fizzy drinks are helpful.
- Sit up straight when eating.
- Do not tackle large lumps of food – cut them up small and chew well.
- Spit out anything not chewed.
- Mix food supplements such as Complan® very thoroughly – dry powder will block the stent.
- If you feel the stent is blocked, stop eating, drink a little and walk around a bit.
- If the blockage persists for more than 3 hours ring your GP or contact the hospital where you were treated.
- Clean the stent after eating with a drink of soda water or lemonade or use this mixture: 4oz sugar, 2oz cream of tartar, 2oz sodium bicarbonate – use one teaspoon of the mixture in a half tumbler of water.
- Keep teeth and dentures in good order so that chewing is effective.

### Foods to avoid:

- Green salads/raw vegetables
- Fried egg white/hard-boiled egg
- Fruit skins and pith of grapefruit and orange
- Tough meat and gristle
- Nuts and dried fruits
- Fish with bones
- White bread, crusty bread, and toast
- Shredded Wheat and Puffed Wheat
- Hard chips and crisps

### Information and support for patients and families:

**Oesophageal Patients' Association** 🖳 www.opa.org.uk
**Cancerbacup** ☎ 0808 800 1234 🖳 www.cancerbacup.org.uk

# Nausea and vomiting

Nausea and vomiting are common symptoms which cause patients and their relatives deep distress. Of the two, nausea causes most misery.

## General principles of management:

- *Assess* – try to identify likely cause—Table 5.5
- *Review medication* – Could medication be the cause? Which antiemetics have been used before and how effective were they?
- *Try non-drug measures* (see below).
- *Choose an antiemetic* – if cause can be identified, choose an antiemetic appropriate for the cause (Table 5.5). Use the antiemetic ladder (Figure 5.3). Administer antiemetics regularly rather than prn and choose an appropriate route of administration (see below).
- *Review frequently* – Is the antiemetic effective? Has the underlying cause of the nausea/vomiting resolved? Avoid changing antiemetic before it has been given an adequate trial at maximum dose.
- ❗ If there is >1 cause of nausea/vomiting you may need >1 drug.

## Route of administration:

- For prophylaxis of nausea and vomiting—use po medication.
- For established nausea or vomiting, consider a parenteral route e.g. syringe driver (📖 p.36 and pp.194–7)—persistent nausea may ↓ gastric emptying and drug absorption. Once symptoms are controlled, consider reverting to a po route.

## Common side effects of antiemetics:

- *Haloperidol and metoclopramide* – restlessness and/or urge to move (akathisia) or parkinsonian effects (e.g. stiffness, tremor).
- *Cyclizine* – anticholinergic effects e.g. dry mouth, blurred vision, urinary retention.
- *Levomepromazine* – sedation at doses >6.25mg b.d.
- *Prokinetic drugs* (e.g. metoclopramide, domperidone) – use with care if bowel obstruction is suspected – may ↑ gut colic/worsen vomiting.
- *Granisetron and ondansetron* – associated with constipation.

## Non-drug measures:
Don't forget non-drug measures to ↓ nausea:
- Avoidance of food smells and unpleasant odours
- Relaxation/diversion/anxiety management
- Acupressure/acupuncture

| Figure 5.3 The antiemetic ladder | | |
|---|---|---|
| **Selected narrow spectrum antiemetic** e.g. <br> • haloperidol *or* <br> • cyclizine *or* <br> • metoclopramide | **2nd-line narrow spectrum** <br> **OR broad spectrum** <br> **OR combination** | e.g. ondansetron <br> e.g. levomepromazine <br> e.g. levomepromazine + ondansetron |

STEP 1  STEP 2

± administer by syringe driver
± dexamethasone

## Table 5.5 Causes of vomiting and choice of antiemetic

| Mechanism of vomiting | Antiemetic |
|---|---|
| Drug/toxin induced or metabolic e.g. hypercalcaemia | Haloperidol (1.5–5mg nocte; particularly for opioid induced vomiting or renal failure). An antiemetic is usually necessary only for the first 4–5d. of opiate therapy |
| | If nausea is persistent and due to opioids, consider changing opioid |
| | Levomepromazine 6.25mg nocte |
| Chemotherapy/ radiotherapy | Granisetron 1mg stat then 1mg bd or ondansetron 8mg bd po or 16mg od pr – particularly for chemotherapy or radiotherapy induced vomiting |
| | Haloperidol 1.5–5mg nocte – for radiotherapy induced vomiting |
| | Dexamethasone 4–8mg daily po or s/cut – often given as part of a chemotherapy regime |
| | Metoclopramide 20mg qds |
| ↑ intracranial pressure | Dexamethasone 4–16mg/d. |
| | Cyclizine 50mg bd/tds (or 150mg/d. via syringe driver) |
| Anxiety, fear or pain | Benzodiazepines e.g. diazepam 2–10mg/d. or midazolam 2.5–5mg stat of 5–20mg subcutaneous infusion |
| | Cyclizine 50mg bd/tds |
| | Levomepromazine 6–25mg/d. |
| Motion/position | Cyclizine 50mg tds po/sc/im |
| | Hyoscine po (300mcgm) or transdermally (1mg/72h.) |
| | Prochlorperazine po (5mg qds) or buccal (3–6mg bd) |
| Gastric stasis* | Domperidone 10mg tds or metoclopramide 10mg tds (particularly if multifactorial with gastric stasis and a central component) |
| Gastric irritation | Stop the irritant if possible e.g. stop NSAIDs |
| | Proton pump inhibitors e.g. lansoprazole 30mg od or omeprazole 20mg od |
| | Antacids |
| | Misoprostol 200mcgm bd – if caused by NSAIDs |
| Constipation | Laxatives/suppositories/enemas |
| Intestinal obstruction | 📖 p.122 |
| Cough induced | 📖 p.138 |
| Unknown cause | Cyclizine 50mg tds or 150mg/d. via syringe driver |
| | Levomepromazine 6–25mg/d. |
| | Dexamethasone 4–8mg daily po/s/cut |
| | Metoclopramide 10–20mg tds/qds po |

* vomits of undigested food without nausea soon after eating

❶ Drugs with antimuscarinic effects (e.g. cyclizine) antagonize prokinetic drugs (e.g. metoclopramide) – if possible, do not use concurrently.

# Dyspepsia

Dyspepsia can be a source of marked morbidity and distress in terminally ill patients.

## Causes[N]:
- Gastro-oesophageal reflux disease (GORD) – 15–25%
- Peptic ulcer (PU) – 15–25%
- Stomach cancer – 2%
- The remaining 60% are classified as *non-ulcer dyspepsia* (NUD, 'functional' dyspepsia)
- *Rare causes:* oesophagitis from swallowed corrosives, oesophageal infection (especially in the immunocompromized)

## Presentation:
- Common symptoms include retrosternal or epigastric pain, fullness, bloating, wind, heartburn, nausea, and vomiting.
- Examination is usually normal – there may be epigastric tenderness.
- Check for clinical anaemia, hepatomegaly, and ascites.

**Differential diagnosis:** Cardiac pain (difficult to distinguish), oesophageal spasm, gallstone pain, pancreatitis, bile reflux.

## Management:
### Lifestyle advice:
- Give advice on healthy eating and smoking cessation.
- Advise patients to avoid precipitating factors e.g. coffee, chocolate, fatty foods.
- Raising the head of the bed and having a main meal well before going to bed may help some people.

### Further measures:
- Avoid or reduce the dose of drugs which cause dyspepsia e.g. potassium supplements, steroids, NSAIDs
- Promote continuing use of antacids/alginates e.g Gaviscon® 10ml qds. Aluminium-containing antacids cause constipation; magnesium-containing antacids are laxative; dimeticone in asilone® is a defoamer, useful for gastric distension/hiccups.
- Try a proton pump inhibitor e.g. lansoprazole 30mg od or omeprazole 20mg od. Treat for 1mo. then stop. If symptoms recur then retreat and after 1mo. reduce dose to a 'maintenance dose' for the long term i.e. lansoprazole 15mg od or omeprazole 10mg od.
- Consider referral for paracentesis if tense ascites
- Consider trying metoclopramide 10mg tds if signs of gastric stasis or distension exist.
- Exclude or treat oesophageal candida – 📖 p.110

## Further information:
**Southwest London and Surrey, West Sussex and Hampshire Cancer Networks** Watson and Lucas. *Adult Palliative Care Guidelines.* 2006.
**NICE** Management of dyspepsia in adults in primary care (2004) 🖥 www.nice.org.uk

## GP Notes: Use of NSAIDs

- All NSAIDs are associated with GI toxicity – risk is ↑ in the elderly. Risks are dose related and vary between drugs.
- Use lower risk NSAIDs e.g. ibuprofen as first-line treatment.
- Start at the lowest recommended dose.
- For the elderly, those on steroids or those with past history of GI ulceration or indigestion, protect the stomach with misoprostol (200mcgms 2–4x/d. taken with the NSAID) or a proton pump inhibitor (PPI e.g. omeprazole 20mg od or lansoprazole 30mg od), or use a COX2 inhibitor (see below).
- Don't use more than one oral NSAID at a time.
- Remember *all* NSAIDs are contraindicated in patients with active peptic ulceration. Non-selective NSAIDs are contraindicated in patients with a history of peptic ulceration.

🚺 Combination of a NSAID and low dose aspirin may ↑ risk of GI side effects: only use this combination if absolutely necessary and if the patient is monitored closely.

🚺 Avoid combination of anticoagulants with NSAIDs – NSAIDs enhance the anticoagulant effect of warfarin and risk of GI bleeding is greatly ↑.

### COX2 inhibitors: COX2 inhibitors:

- Have NO effect on platelet aggregation.
- Have no benefit over non-selective NSAIDs if used in patients on continuous low-dose aspirin, *and*
- Combining a COX2 inhibitor with PPI/misoprostol does NOT give extra stomach protection.

⚠ Due to concerns about cardiovascular safety, *only* use COX2 inhibitors in preference to standard NSAIDs when specifically indicated (i.e. for patients at high risk of developing gastroduodenal ulcer, perforation, or bleeding) and after an assessment of cardiovascular risk. Switch patients receiving a COX2 inhibitor who have ischaemic heart disease or cerebrovascular disease to alternative treatment.

# Gastrointestinal (GI) bleeding

**Causes:** Box 5.3. Bleeding due to cancer is usually due to a primary carcinoma of the stomach, oesophagus, or colon.

**Risk factors:** NSAIDs, steroids, anticoagulation, excess alcohol consumption, liver disease.

## Presentation:

**Upper GI bleeding:** *Typical presentation:*
- Haematemesis – vomiting of blood
- Melaena – passage of black, offensive, tarry stool consisting of digested blood per rectum

🛈 Iron tablets may cause black stools.

**Lower GI bleeding:** *Typical presentation:*
- Passage of fresh blood PR.

🛈 Very heavy upper GI bleeds can present with fresh red bleeding PR.

**Other features that may be present:**
- Faintness or dizziness especially on standing
- Patient feels cold or clammy
- Collapse ± cardiac arrest

## Examination:
- Pulse – tachycardia
- BP – ↓ and/or postural drop
- JVP – ↓
- Vomitus

## Management:

---

**Severe, life-threatening bleed:** Make a decision whether the cause of the bleed is treatable or a terminal event. This is best done in advance but bleeding can't always be predicted. 🛈 Palliative treatment options include laser treatment and arterial embolization – both can be performed on frail patients.

- **Severe bleed – active treatment**: Briefly assess the severity of the bleed from history and examination (or history alone if based on telephone information). If a significant bleed is suspected:
  - Call for emergency ambulance support
  - Lie the patient flat and lift legs higher than body (e.g. feet on pillow)
  - Insert a large-bore IV cannula – the opportunity may be lost by the time the ambulance crew arrive. If possible take a sample for FBC and X-match on insertion.
  - If available, give oxygen.
  - If available, start plasma expander/IV fluids.
  - Transfer as rapidly as possible to hospital.
- **Severe bleed – no active treatment:**
  - Stay with the patient
  - Give sedative medication e.g. midazolam 10–40mg s/cut or slow IV or diazepam 10–20mg pr and diamorphine 5–10mg s/cut or IV if in pain
  - Support carers as major bleeds are extremely distressing.

**Non-life threatening bleed:** Unless the patient is very frail, admit for further investigation. Occasionally small bleeds herald much larger ones.

*If acute admission is not appropriate:* Reassure, monitor frequently. Follow up is directed at cause:
- Check FBC and clotting screen – if on anticoagulants or there is a possible bleeding tendency. Consider addressing clotting problem and/or iron supplements or transfusion (🕮 p.106).
- Treat infection that might exacerbate a bleed.
- Consider minimizing bleeding tendency with tranexamic acid 1g tds po – stop if no effect after 1wk. If effective, continue for 1wk. after bleeding has stopped. Continue 500mg tds long-term if bleeding recurs and responds to a further course of treatment. Weigh up benefits of stopping bleeding against ↑ risk of stroke or MI.
- Etamsylate 500mg qds can be useful for capillary bleeding.
- Upper GI bleeding – stop NSAIDs, start PPI e.g. omeprazole 20mg od or lansoprazole 30mg od ± consider referral for gastroscopy.
- Lower GI bleeding – consider rectal steroids to ↓ inflammation or rectal tranexamic acid ± referral for colonoscopy. Oral sucralfate has been used for post-radiation proctitis (applied topically pr).
- Referral for radiotherapy (if bleeding from tumour), chemotherapy, or palliative surgery (e.g. cautery) is an option in some cases.

---

### Box 5.3 Causes of GI bleeding

**Upper GI bleed:**
- Peptic ulcer
- Gastritis
- Mallory-Weiss tear
- Oesophagitis
- Oesophageal or gastric cancer
- Oesophageal varices
- Drugs – NSAIDs, steroids, anticoagulants
- Angiodysplasia
- Haemangioma
- Bleeding disorders
- Swallowed blood from nosebleed

**Lower GI bleed:**
- Diverticulitis
- Colitis – infectious or inflammatory
- Large bowel tumour or polyp
- Haemorrhoids
- Anal fissure
- Angiodysplasia (arterio-venous malformations are common)
- Haemangioma
- Bleeding disorders
- Blood from upper GI bleed

---

### GP Notes:

ⓘ In all patients likely to bleed, consider pre-warning carers and giving them a strategy. Risks of frightening a family with information about possible catastrophic haemoptysis need to be balanced against potential distress that could be caused by leaving a patient and family unprepared.

# Constipation

Constipation is the passage of hard stools less frequently than the patient's own normal pattern. It is a very common symptom.

**Causes:** Box 5.4

**Assessment:** Stool frequency varies considerably.

- *Establish symptoms and onset.* What is normal for the patient? What does the patient mean by constipation? Is this symptom a recent change? When did s/he last have a bowel movement? Was the stool normal for him/her? Specifically ask about tenesmus, blood in stool, abdominal pain, and diarrhoea.
- *Check current medication:* Does the patient use laxatives? If so, which ones and how often?
- *Background information:* ask about diet
- *Examine the abdomen:* for masses and hepatomegaly. Rectal examination is essential to exclude a low rectal or anal tumour obstructing the bowel and detect faecal impaction.
- *Consider checking U&E, Ca²⁺ and thyroid function tests:* only check if you intend to treat if an abnormality is found.

⚠ Constipation can herald spinal cord compression (📖 p.149). If suspected, undertake a full neurological examination.

**Occult presentations:** Common in the very elderly and frail. *Include:*

- Confusion
- Urinary retention
- Abdominal pain
- Overflow diarrhoea
- Loss of appetite
- Nausea and/or vomiting

## Management:

- Pre-empt constipation by putting everyone at risk (e.g. patients on opioids) on regular laxatives.
- Treat reversible causes e.g. give analgesia if pain on defaecation, alter diet, ↑ fluid intake.
- Treat with regular stool softener (e.g. lactulose) ± regular bowel stimulant (e.g. senna) or alternatively use a combination drug (e.g. co-danthrusate). Titrate dose against reponse. The aim of laxative therapy is to promote comfortable defaecation – not increase frequency.
- If that is ineffective, consider adding rectal measures. Ask – Is the rectum full? Is the stool soft or hard?
  - Soft stools and lax rectum – try bisacodyl suppositories (🚫 must come into direct contact with rectum).
  - Hard stools – try glycerol suppositories – insert into the faeces and allow to dissolve. Softener and rectal stimulant – acts in 1–6h.
- If still not cleared, refer to the district nurse for lubricant ± high phosphate (stimulant) enema (usually act in ~20min.).
- Once cleared, leave on a regular aperient with instructions to ↑ aperients if constipation recurs.

**Manual evacuation:** May occasionally be necessary. Liaise closely with nursing staff. Do not attempt without some form of sedation or analgesia. Consent is an important and necessary part of this procedure.

## Box 5.4 Causes of constipation

| Malignancy | Colonic, ovarian, and uterine tumours |
|---|---|
| Pain | Anal fissure, perianal abscess |
| Benign colorectal disease | Diverticular disease, distal proctitis, anterior mucosal prolapse, benign stricture, intussusception, volvulus. |
| Endocrine/ metabolic | Hypercalcaemia, hypothyroidism, DM with autonomic neuropathy |
| Drugs | Opioids, antacids containing calcium or aluminium, antidepressants, iron, diuretics, antiparkinsonian medication, antimuscarinics e.g. phenothiazines, hyoscine, octreotide, anticonvulsants, antihistamines, calcium antagonists. |
| Other | Immobility, weakness (inability to ↑ intra-abdominal pressure), old age, poor diet, poor fluid intake, ↑ fluid loss (e.g. vomiting, diarrhoea, fever) |

## Table 5.6 Drugs commonly used to treat constipation (BNF 1.6)

| Laxative | Comments | Speed of action |
|---|---|---|
| Bulk forming e.g. bran, ispaghula, sterculia Methylcellulose is bulk forming and a softener | ↑ faecal mass and stimulate peristalsis Useful for patients with small, hard stools where dietary fibre can't be ↑ Maintain fluid intake >1l/d. to avoid bowel obstruction | Full effect takes several days to develop |
| Stimulant e.g. senna (7.5–30mg nocte), bisacodyl (5–10mg nocte) Docusate acts as stimulant and softener | ↑ intestinal motility Often cause abdominal cramp Avoid in intestinal obstruction | Senna – 8–12h. Bisacodyl • tablets – 10–12h. • suppositories – 20–60min. |
| Lubricant/softening e.g. docusate (up to 500mg/d. in divided doses) | Surfactant action draws water into the stool | 1–2 days |
| Osmotic e.g. lactulose, magnesium hydroxide (25–50ml prn), macrogols (Movicol® 1–3 sachets/d. in divided doses) | ↑ water in the large bowel Dehydrating so maintain fluid intake >1l/d. May cause abdominal distention/cramps | Lactulose—48h. Macrogols—1–2d. |
| Combination e.g. co-danthramer (dantron + poloxamer '188', 1–2 capsules nocte); co-danthrusate (dantron + docusate, 1–3 capsules nocte) | Dantron is a stimulant laxative. Use of dantron is limited to the very elderly and those with terminal illness as it is carcinogenic in rats May colour urine red Avoid if incontinence as is a skin irritant | 6–12h. |

# Other GI problems

**Ascites:** Free fluid in the peritoneal cavity.

**Presentation:** abdominal distention. Examination reveals shifting dullness to percussion ± fluid thrill.

*Causes:* Box 5.5

**Management:** Depending on clinical state consider referring for radio- or chemotherapy if appropriate *or* treat symptoms:
- Give analgesia for discomfort.
- Refer for paracentesis and/or peritoneo-venous shunt (if recurrent ascites) if the patient is well enough. ❗ Shunts frequently block.
- Try diuretics – furosemide 20–40mg od and/or spironolactone 100–600mg od. May take a week to produce maximal effect. More likely to be useful if the patient has liver metastases causing hepatic dysfunction. ❗ Monitor albumin level – if low, diuretics make ascites worse.
- Dexamethasone 2–4mg/d. may help – discontinue if not effective.
- Try support stockings and/or massage for leg oedema.
- 'Squashed stomach syndrome' – try prokinetics e.g. domperidone or metoclopramide 10mg tds.

> ⚠ Most patients with malignancy-related ascites have poor prognosis – a principle of minimal disturbance should usually guide management.

**Obstruction/subacute obstruction of the bowel:** Often of complex origin with functional and mechanical elements.

**Presentation:**
- Vomiting – often faeculent with little preceding nausea
- Constipation
- Abdominal distention
- Examination reveals an empty rectum

**Treatment options:**

*Active treatment:*
- If surgery is an option, then refer for a surgical opinion
- If the patient is otherwise well, consider referral to an oncologist – ovarian and colonic cancers often respond to chemotherapy.

*Symptomatic treatment:* If active treatment is not an option:
- Keep the patient hydrated stool soft.
- Dexamethasone 4–8mg/d. is antiemetic and minimizes obstruction.
- If colic is a problem, stop prokinetics (metoclopramide/domperidone) and start an antispasmodic (e.g. hyoscine 300mcgm tds po).
- For pain, give an opioid—via syringe driver if risk of malabsorption.
- Aim to abolish nausea and keep vomiting to a minimum (may be impossible to abolish vomiting) with cyclizine, haloperidol or levomepromazine. If vomiting can't be controlled, consider referral for venting gastrostomy.
- Consider referral to palliative care for antisecretory agents (e.g. octreotide). ❗ Octreotide dries up all GI secretions tending towards constipation.

## Box 5.5 Causes of ascites

- Malignancy – any intra-abdominal organ, ovary (50% patients with ovarian cancer have ascites) or kidney – often indicative of end-stage disease.
- Hypoproteinaemia e.g. nephrotic syndrome, renal failure.
- Right heart failure.
- Portal hypertension.

## Further information:

**European Journal of Palliative Care** Campbell C *Controlling malignant ascites* (2001). **8**(5): 187–91.

**Palliative Medicine** Stephenson & Gilbert *The development of clinical guidelines on paracentesis for ascites related to malignancy* (2002). **16**(3): 213–8.

**BMJ** Baines M *ABC of palliative care: Nausea, vomiting and intestinal obstruction* (1997). **315**: 1148–50. ⊞ www.bmj.com

**Gut fistulae:** Connections from the gut to other organs – commonly skin, bladder, or vagina. Bowel fistulae are characterized by air passing through the fistula channel.

**Management:**
- If well enough for surgery, refer to a surgeon.
- If not fit for surgery consider referring to palliative care for octreotide.

**Diarrhoea:** Defined as passage of ≥3 loose stools/d. Clarify what the patient/carer means by diarrhoea. Less common than constipation but can be distressing for the patient and difficult for the carer – especially if incontinence results.

**Management:**
- ↑ fluid intake – small amounts of clear fluids frequently.
- Screen for infection (including pseudomembranous colitis if diarrhoea after a course of antibiotics) and treat if necessary.
- Ensure no overflow diarrhoea 2° to constipation.
- Ensure no excessive/erratic laxative use.
- Ensure no other medication is causing diarrhoea.
- Consider giving aspirin (300–600mg tds) – ↓ intestinal electrolyte and water secretion caused by prostaglandins. May particularly help with radiation-induced diarrhoea.
- Consider ondansetron 4mg tds for radiotherapy-induced diarrhoea.
- Consider giving pancreatic enzyme supplements e.g. creon® 25000 tds prior to meals if fat malabsorption (e.g. 2° to pancreatic carcinoma).
- Otherwise treat symptomatically with codeine phosphate 30–60mg qds or loperamide 2mg tds/qds.
- Refer to palliative care if unable to control symptoms.

**Tenesmus:** Sensation in the rectum of incomplete emptying following defaecation – as if there is something left behind which cannot be passed. It is most common in association with irritable bowel syndrome, but can be caused by tumour.

**Management:**
- Prevent and treat constipation (📖 p.120)
- Give analgesia
- NSAID e.g. diclofenac 50mg tds
- Opioids – variable effect
- Neuropathic painkillers e.g. amitriptyline or anticonvulsants
- Nifedipine 10–20mg bd, nitrates or baclofen may help due to their effect on muscle tone
- Steroids may be helpful

Depending on clinical state and cause of tenesmus, consider referral for radiotherapy (if the cause is a tumour), lumbar sympathectomy (>80% success rate) or spinal infusion of local anaesthetic ± opioids.

## GP Notes: Diagnosing cause of diarrhoea

- Defaecation described as 'diarrhoea' happening only 2–3x/d. without warning suggests anal incontinence.
- Profuse watery stools are characteristic of colonic diarrhoea.
- Sudden onset of diarrhoea after a period of constipation raises suspicion of faecal impaction and 'overflow' diarrhoea.
- Alternating diarrhoea and constipation suggests poorly regulated laxative therapy or impending bowel obstruction.
- Pale, fatty, offensive stools (steatorrhoea) indicate malabsorption due to either pancreatic or ileal disease.

**Further information:**

**Doyle** *et al. Oxford Textbook of Palliative Medicine.* (2005). OUP. ISBN: 0198566980.

# Patients with ostomies

The first iatrogenic stoma was constructed in France in 1776 for an obstructing rectal cancer. Stomas (from the Greek meaning 'mouth') may be temporary (de-functioning) or permanent.

## Common problems:

**Psycho-social problems:** Self-help groups provide information and tips on lifestyle and stoma care; specialist stoma nurses can provide support and counselling.

**Stoma retraction:** Can cause leakage and severe skin problems. Most common reason for re-operation. Refer for specialist advice.

**Prolapse:** Seen most frequently with loop colostomy. If persists and disrupts pouching, refer for consideration of revision.

**Peristomal hernia:** Common complication. Symptomatic cases require referral for repair unless life expectancy is very limited.

**Stenosis:** Narrowing of the stoma may result in difficulty or pain passing stool and/or obstruction. If problematic, refer for revision.

**Skin complications:** Skin irritation can be due to:
- Leakage onto the skin
- Allergic reactions to the adhesive material in a skin barrier
- Fungal infection
- Inadequate hygiene

**Drugs:** Enteric-coated and modified release preparations are unsuitable for people with bowel stomas – particularly for patients with ileostomy.

**Diet:**
- Avoid foods that cause intestinal upset or diarrhoea.
- In the case of descending/sigmoid colostomy, avoid foods that cause constipation. If constipated, ↑ fluid intake and/or dietary fibre.
- Certain foods e.g. beans, cucumbers, and carbonated drinks can cause gas, as can certain habits such as talking or swallowing air while eating, using straws, mouth breathing, and chewing gum.
- A daily portion of apple sauce, cranberry juice, yogurt, or buttermilk can help control odour. If odour is strong and persistent, consider use of charcoal filters.

**Activities:** Advise patients to avoid rough contact sports and heavy lifting as these might lead to herniation around the stoma. Patients with stomas may swim. Water will not enter a stoma due to peristalsis so stomas do not need to be covered when bathing.

**Travel:** Advise patients to pack sufficient supplies of their stoma products and carry supplies with them in case baggage is misplaced. Avoid storing supplies in a very hot environment as heat may damage pouches.

🛈 In all cases liaise with a specialist stoma nurse if possible.

## Table 5.7 The three main types of stoma

|  | Colostomy | Ileostomy | Urostomy |
|---|---|---|---|
| Output | Depends on site:<br>• transverse colostomy—soft stool<br>• descending/sigmoid colostomy—formed stool | Soft/fluid stool | Urine – continent procedures using bowel to fashion a bladder which is then drained with a catheter through the stoma are becoming common |
| Reasons for using this type of stoma | Carcinoma<br>Diverticular disease<br>Trauma<br>Radiation enteritis<br>Bowel ischaemia<br>Hirschprung's disease<br>Congenital abnormalities<br>Obstruction<br>Crohn's disease<br>Faecal incontinence | Ulcerative colitis<br>Crohn's disease<br>Familial polyposis coli<br>Obstruction<br>Radiation enteritis<br>Trauma<br>Bowel ischaemia<br>Carcinoma | Carcinoma<br>Urinary incontinence<br>Fistulae<br>Spinal column disorders |

### GP Notes: Prevention of skin complications

- Advise patients to clean, rinse, and pat the skin dry between pouch changes.
- Advise patients to avoid using an oily soap, which can leave a film that interferes with proper adhesion of the skin barrier.
- Ensure the pouch system fits.
- Treat any infection with oral antibiotics and/or oral/topical antifungals.
- Apply skin barrier cream.
- If the skin is uneven (e.g. due to scarring), fill irregularities with stoma paste to give a better fit.
- Consider the use of convex discs or stoma belts (refer to specialist stoma nurse for advice).

127

### Advice for patients: Information and support for patients and carers

British Colostomy Association ☎ 0800 328 4257
🖳 www.colostomyassociation.org.uk

# Incontinence of urine

Urinary incontinence in advanced illness can be a cause of great embarrassment to patients and carers and also cause an increased sense of isolation. Active management of the symptom can bring great comfort to the patient and their family.

## Presentation:

**History:** A good history is essential to establish the likely cause and so direct management decisions appropriately.

- Frequency of complaint
- Degree of incapacity
- Whether occurs with standing/coughing/sneezing
- Urgency/dysuria/frequency of micturition
- Volume passed
- Past obstetric and medical history
- Medication
- Mobility
- Accessibility of toilets

## Examination:

- *Abdominal including rectal examination* – enlarged bladder, masses, loaded colon, faecal impaction, anal tone.
- *Pelvic* – prolapse, atrophy, neurological deficit, retention of urine, and pelvic masses.

**Investigation:** Intake/output diary – evaluates problem and benchmark for progress (record drinks and passage of urine); Urine – glucose, RBCs, MC&S; consider U&E/fasting blood glucose if renal impairment or DM is suspected.

🛈 Patients may have a mixed pattern of incontinence.

## Drugs that exacerbate/cause incontinence: Diuretics, antihistamines, anxiolytics, α-blockers, sedatives and hypnotics, anticholinergic drugs, tricyclic antidepressants.

## General measures:

- Manipulate fluid intake – amount, type (avoid tea, coffee, alcohol), timing of fluids at night.
- Alter medication e.g. timing of diuretics.
- Treat UTI and chronic respiratory conditions.
- Avoid constipation.
- Consider HRT (topical or systemic) for oestrogen deficiency.

**Functional incontinence:** No urological problem. Caused by other factors e.g. inaccessible toilets/immobility, behavioural problems, cognitive deficit. Treat the cause.

## Total urethral incontinence:

- *Symptoms:* Uncontrollable loss of urine.
- *Causes:* Incompetence of the urethral sphincter (e.g. due to tumour invasion or surgical intervention) or central loss of sphincter control (e.g. due to confusion or dementia).
- *Treatment:* Incontinence aids e.g. pads or catheters. If the cause is central loss of sphincter control, regular toileting may be effective.

## GP Notes: Aids and appliances for incontinence

**Pads:** Many different types. DNs or continence advisors are best aware of those available via the NHS locally. They are not prescribable on FP10 and supplied by local NHS Trusts on a 'daily allowance' basis. This situation varies across the country.

**Bed covers:** Absorb 1–4l of urine. Good laundry facilities are needed. If left wet, can cause skin breakdown. Available via NHS Trusts.

**External catheters or sheaths/conveens:** Can be prescribed on NHS prescription. Approved appliances are listed in part IXB of the UK Drug Tariff. Used for men who have intractable incontinence and who are highly physically dependent, do not have urine retention and do not require an internal catheter. Assessment and fitting by a DN or continence adviser is essential. Used in association with a drainage bag. *Types:*
- Self-adhesive e.g. Bard (Integrity) or attached with adhesive strips e.g. NorthWest Medical (Uridrop and Uristrip). Adhesive sheaths can last several days but daily changing is recommended.
- Non-adhesive e.g. Manfred Sauer (Comfort sheath). Replace non-adhesive sheaths 2–3x/d.. Some are reusable e.g. Bard (Urosheath).

*Problems:* Include ↑ susceptibility to UTI, sores on penis and skin irritation due to the adhesive.

**Indwelling catheters:** 📖 p.131

**Intermittent self-catheterization:** The patient inserts a catheter into his/her bladder 4–5x/d. to drain urine. ↓ problems of infection and blockage. Useful for neurological bladder dysfunction. *Types:*
- *Reusable silver or stainless steel* e.g. Malvern (Biscath®)
- *Reusable PVC* e.g. Bard (Reliacath®), Rüsch (Riplex®) – can be washed and reused for 1wk. Usually supply 5/mo.
- *Single use* e.g. Astra Tech (Lofric®) – need 125–150/mo. Expensive. Only use on consultant advice.

**Collecting bags:** Can be prescribed on NHS prescription. Approved appliances are listed in part IXB of the UK Drug Tariff.
- *Leg bags:* Drainable bags last 5–7d.. Usually 500/750mls e.g. Bard (Uriplan®). Larger capacity bags are too heavy for mobile patients. A variety of attachment systems are available on prescription. Long tubes are needed to wear a bag on the calf.
- *Night drainage bags:* Connect to night bag attachment of day bags. Single use, non-draining bags are recommended e.g. Coloplast (Simpla S2®), Bard (Uriplan®). Bag hangers are not available on FP10.

**Urostomy:** 📖 p.126

## Further information:

**PPA.** Electronic drug tariff 🖥 www.ppa.org.uk
**Association for Continence Advice.** Advice for health care professionals 🖥 www.aca.uk.com

**Neurological incontinence:** Bladder function is a reflex action we learn to override as children.
- If a lesion is above T6 level, automatic emptying will occur when the bladder is full – though there is no control.
- If the lesion is below this level (e.g. damage to sacral plexus or lower spinal cord/cauda equine compression) there is no emptying reflex.

Usually, catheterization is needed – though, depending on the level of the lesion and manual dexterity of the patient, intermittent self-catheterization might be an option. Anticholinergics can help.

### Stress incontinence:
- *Symptoms:* Small losses of urine without warning throughout the day related to coughing/exercise.
- *Causes:* Prostatectomy; childbirth; ageing.
- *Treatment:* Pelvic floor exercises help 60% (taught by physiotherapists/ continence advisors; leaflets available). Mechanical devices (e.g. Conveen continence guard®) help 75%. Ring pessaries are helpful for associated prolapse but do not usually control incontinence.

**Urge incontinence:** Detrusor instability or hyperreflexia cause the bladder to contract unintentionally.
- *Symptoms:* Frequency, overwhelming desire to void (often precipitated by stressful event), large loss, nocturia.
- *Causes:* Idiopathic, neurological problems (e.g. stroke, MS), local irritation (bladder stones, infection), obstruction (benign prostatic hypertrophy), surgery (transurethral resection of the prostate).
- *Treatment:* Try bladder training programmes – resist the urge to pass urine for increasing periods. Start with an achievable interval based on diary evidence and ↑ slowly. Drugs are helpful e.g. oxybutynin, amitriptyline (nocturnal symptoms). Spontaneously remits/relapses so reassess every 3–4mo.

### Overflow:
- *Symptoms:* Constant dribbling loss day and night.
- *Causes:* Benign prostatic hypertrophy, prostate cancer, urethral stricture, faecal impaction, neurological (lower motor neurone lesions), side effect of medication.
- *Treatment:* Aimed at relieving the obstruction – treatment of constipation, catheterization, surgery.

**Urinary fistula:** Communication between bladder and the outside – normally through vagina. Results in constant dribbling loss day and night.
- *Causes:* Congenital, malignancy, complication of surgery.
- *Treatment:* Consider referral to gynaecology/urology depending on the clinical state of the patient. Protection of the skin is paramount, using barrier creams or sprays.

130

---

### Advice for patients: Information and support

**Bladder and Bowel Foundation** ☎ 0845 345 0165
🖥 www.bladderandbowelfoundation.org
**Spinal Injuries Association** ☎ 0845 678 6633 🖥 www.spinal.co.uk

## GP Notes: Indwelling catheters

Can be prescribed on NHS prescription. Approved appliances are listed in part IXA of the UK Drug Tariff. Only use catheters in patients with urinary retention, incontinence, or problems getting to the toilet (e.g. bed bound).

**Types:** Only long-term Foley catheters are suitable for use in primary care. They last 3–12wk. (usually change every 6wk.).
* Hydrogel coated: e.g. Bard (Biocath®)
* Silicone elastomer: Coated latex e.g. Bard, Rüsch (Sympacath®)
* All silicone: e.g. Coloplast, Medasil, Rüsch (Brilliant Aquaflate®)

**Catheter size:** Unless specified a 12 or 14Ch catheter is supplied. Use smallest diameter of catheter that drains urine effectively. Catheters >16Ch are more likely to cause bypassing of urine around the catheter and urethral strictures but may be needed if there is a lot of bladder debris or clot retention.

**Catheter length:** Men require longer catheters than women. Specify 'male' or 'female' on the prescription.

**Catheter balloon:** 10ml balloons are supplied unless specified otherwise. Pre-filled catheters contain sterile water which inflates the retaining balloon with water. They are more expensive but quicker to insert and there are no costs for syringes or sterile water.

**Drainage:** Usually attached to a leg bag though catheter valves are also available allowing the patient to use his/her bladder as a urine reservoir. The valve must be released every 3–4h.to drain out the urine.

### Table 5.8 Common catheter problems

| | |
|---|---|
| Leakage | Check if constipated or catheter blocked. Try smaller gauge catheter. Use skin barrier creams to prevent skin problems. |
| Infection | 90% develop bacteriuria <4 wk. after insertion. Always confirm suspected UTI with MSU – only treat if symptomatic or Proteus species grown. May prove difficult to eliminate. |
| Encrustation | Deposition from the urine onto the catheter. May cause catheter blockage or pain on changing catheter. Check urine pH regularly in patients with problems. Citric acid patency solutions may help if pH >7.4. Alternatively try a daily dose of vitamin C. |
| Inflammation | Due to presence of a catheter in the urethra. Exacerbated by encrustation and infection. Remove secretions/crusting with soap and water. If inflammation continues, try a different catheter type. |
| Blockage | Flush the catheter with normal saline or 0.02% chlorhexidine. If unsuccessful, change catheter. Alter the interval of routine changes if regular blockage towards the end of catheter-life. |
| Bladder spasm | Irritation of the trigone of the bladder. Remove some water from the balloon (though catheter may fall out). Antispasmodics (e.g. oxybutynin) may help. Consider referral for suprapubic catheter. |

*Unable to insert catheter, deflate balloon to remove catheter, or false passage formation* – Refer to urology

# Haematuria

Haematuria ranges from microscopic haematuria discovered incidentally on urinalysis, to frank haematuria with the passage of clots ± clot retention. The amount of bleeding does not always correlate with severity of cause.

ⓘ Urine discolouration, which can be confused with haematuria, can result from:
- Beetroot ingestion
- Porphyria and
- Certain drugs (e.g. rifampicin, co-danthramer)

**Causes:** Box 5.6

**Investigations:** Urine infection is uncomfortable and not usually a terminal event. Always investigate urine with M, C&S to exclude urine infection, unless the patient is very close to death.

Appropriateness of other investigations depends on the clinical state of the patient. Don't investigate if you don't intend to treat.

### Other possible investigations include:
- Renal/bladder USS
- Intravenous urography – to look for obstructive lesions and stones
- Referral for cystoscopy

### Management:
- ↑ fluid intake to promote good urine output (helps avoid clot retention and clear UTI).
- Treat reversible causes e.g. UTI, bleeding tendency.
- Stop drugs which might be causing/exacerbating bleeding.
- If anaemic, consider iron supplements or transfusion.
- Etamsylate 500mg qds may help by ↓ capillary bleeding in the bladder.
- Consider referral for palliative radiotherapy.
- Bleeding from the prostate may respond to finasteride 5mg od.
- If severe bleeding, which is not a terminal event, consider admission for iliac artery embolization.

☛ Use of tranexamic acid is controversial – it may cause formation of hard clots which then need to be irrigated cystoscopically.

**Clot retention:** Needs specialist management – admit. Specialist care involves evacuation of bladder clots. A non-distended bladder bleeds far less than a distended bladder.

## Box 5.6 Causes of haematuria

- Kidney – tumour, stones, infection, glomerulonephritis.
- Ureter – tumour, stones.
- Bladder – tumour, infection, stones, chronic inflammation, drug-induced haemorrhagic cystitis (caused by cyclophosphamide and ifosfamide).
- Prostate – prostatitis, tumour (post-radiotherapy or locally advanced tumour).
- Urethra – inflammation.
- Gynaecological – menstruation, postmenopausal bleeding, cervical bleeding, atrophic vaginitis.
- Systemic clotting disorder – there is usually evidence of bruising or bleeding elsewhere too.
- Aspirin and NSAIDs don't usually cause haematuria but bleeding associated with surgical interventions may be exacerbated/prolonged.

🚨 Free Hb and myoglobin make urine test sticks +ve in absence of red cells.

# Sexual health in advanced disease

Discussion of sexual issues is important but patients often find it difficult to ask for help as they are embarrassed and assume nothing can be done. Healthcare professionals also find it a difficult area to talk about both due to their own inhibitions and because they don't think they have the knowledge to deal with problems.

**Facts:**
- Individuals with advanced cancer often remain sexually active.
- Problems that arise may be physical, psychological or due to relationship changes and there are frequently several factors involved.
- Many sexual problems are solvable.

🛈 Patients or partners of patients with cancer may fear that cancer can be transmitted through sex.

**General issues:** Lack of libido in both sexes can be caused by:
- Change in body image e.g. surgery, disfigurement, presence of stoma
- Depression
- Relationship problems
- Hormone deficiency — male and female
- Drug-related side-effects
- Physical problems such as breathlessness, weakness, and pain

**Management:**
- Explore sexual issues with open questions e.g. Has your disease affected the way you view yourself? Has it affected your relationships? Allow the patient to guide the consultation into more specific areas.
- Address specific symptoms e.g. breathlessness.
- Loss of libido postmenopause responds to administration of androgens e.g. testosterone implants in combination with HRT until libido is re-established. If the patient has a gynaecological or breast cancer, do not prescribe hormones without seeking specialist advice.
- Consider referral to specialist counsellor for further support.

**Dyspareunia:** Common symptom in women. May be caused by
- *Fear of pain on intercourse* e.g. due to pelvic surgery. Can cause tensing of the vaginal muscles (vaginismus) and pain on intercourse. Reassure. If not improving refer for specialist counselling.
- *Vaginal dryness* — most commonly due to lack of oestrogen or fear. May also be due to radiotherapy. Advise vaginal lubricants. Consider a trial of topical oestrogen (e.g. estradiol tablet 25mcgm nocte for 2wk. then twice weekly for 3mo.) or HRT.
- *Vaginal soreness* — check for infection, Thrush is the commonest cause. Treat with topical imidazole pessaries e.g. clotrimazole 500mg nocte x1 ± cream or fluconazole 150mg x 1. If no response, send swabs for M, C&S. Topical lidocaine gel can be helpful if no cause is found.
- *Vaginal stenosis* e.g. following surgery or radiotherapy. Refer for expert advice. Treatment is with vaginal dilators ± surgery.
- *Chronic pelvic pain* — may be caused by underlying disease or as a result of treatment of the underlying disease (e.g. surgery or radiotherapy). If cause is untreatable, limiting penetration may help.

## Table 5.9 Drugs associated with sexual dysfunction

| Endocrine drugs: | Antihypertensives: |
|---|---|
| • Antiandrogens e.g. cyproterone acetate<br>• Anti-oestrogens e.g. tamoxifen (↓ libido in women)<br>• Gonadorelin analogues e.g. goserelin implants | • Thiazide diuretics e.g. bendroflumethiazide<br>• β-blockers e.g. atenolol |
| Psychotropic drugs: | Others: |
| • Antidepressants e.g. SSRIs<br>• Phenothiazines e.g. levomepromazine<br>• Butyrophenones e.g. haloperidol<br>• Anxiolytics/hypnotics e.g. diazepam | • Alcohol<br>• Recreational drugs<br>• Digoxin<br>• Spironolactone<br>• Ranitidine<br>• Metoclopramide<br>• Carbamazepine |

### Advice for patients: Patient experience

'When my partner developed bowel cancer every health care professional chose to assume that we were no longer sexually intimate. Not one professional raised the matter with us and we were left on our own to struggle through the guilts and practicalities of maintaining this very important aspect of our lives just when we needed to affirm each other most.'

### Further information:

**Tomlinson J** *ABC of Sexual Health* (1999). BMJ Publishing. ISBN: 0727917595.
**Nursing Times** Law C Sexual health and the respiratory patient (2001). **97:** NT Plus XI–XII.
**Oncologist** Penson *et al.* Sexuality and cancer: conversation comfort zone (2000). **5:** 336–44.

**Erectile dysfunction (impotence):** Persistent inability to obtain or maintain sufficient rigidity of the penis to allow satisfactory sexual performance.
- Drug causes (Table 5.9, 📖 p.135).
- Disease/treatment effects – spinal cord compression, pelvic malignancy, pelvic surgery/radiotherapy, orchidectomy, brain neoplasm.
- Concurrent disease – DM, peripheral vascular disease, age-related.
- Psychological – fear of failure to acquire or maintain an erection or fear of experiencing or causing pain.

**Management:** Figure 5.4
- Review medication – stop or change any drugs that might be causing the problem.
- Phosphodiesterase type 5 inhibitors (PDE5s) are the mainstays of treatment – titrate dose to effect (most diabetics need the maximum dose); warn the patient he may need around 8 attempts before a satisfactory erection occurs; side effects include headache, flushing and acid reflux.
- Review progress – adjust dosage and/or consider other treatment options – intraurethral/intracavernosal alprostadil or vacuum devices may rarely be appropriate for selected patients – refer to urology.

| Table 5.10 PDE5 inhibitors and action times | | | |
|---|---|---|---|
| **Drug** | **Onset of action in min. (*Peak action*)** | **Duration of action (h.)** | **Doses** |
| Sildenafil | 20–30 (*60*) | 4–6 | 25–50–100mg |
| Tadalafil | 60–120 (*120*) | 36–48 | 10–20mg |
| Vardenafil | 20–30 (*60*) | 4–6 | 5–10–20mg |
| ⚠ PDE5 inhibitors are contraindicated for patients taking nicorandil or nitrates, or immediately after MI or stroke. | | | |
| Reproduced with permission from British Heart Foundation factfile: Drugs for erectile dysfunction (6/2005) available from 🖳 www.bhf.org.uk | | | |

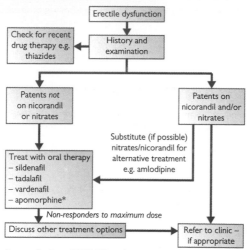

**Figure 5.4 Algorithm for the management of erectile dysfunction**

Erectile dysfunction → History and examination

Check for recent drug therapy e.g. thiazides

Patents *not* on nicorandil or nitrates

Patents on nicorandil and/or nitrates

Substitute (if possible) nitrates/nicorandil for alternative treatment e.g. amlodipine

Treat with oral therapy
– sildenafil
– tadalafil
– vardenafil
– apomorphine*

*Non-responders to maximum dose*

Discuss other treatment options

Refer to clinic – if appropriate

*not as effective as PDE5 inhibitors but not contraindicated with nitrates.

Reproduced in modified form with permission from British Heart Foundation fact file: Drugs for erectile dysfunction (6/2005) available from ⌨ www.bhf.org.uk

**GP Notes:**

❶ NHS prescriptions for impotence are available **only** for men:
- Treated for prostate cancer; with kidney failure, spinal cord injury, DM, MS, spina bifida, Parkinson's disease, polio, severe pelvic injury or who have had radical pelvic surgery or a prostatectomy.
- Already receiving drug treatment for impotence on 14.9.98
- Through specialist services for men suffering severe distress due to impotence.

Endorse FP10/GP10 with SLS.

# Stridor and cough

**Stridor:** Coarse wheezing sound that results from the obstruction of a major airway e.g. larynx.

**Management:**
- Corticosteroids (e.g. dexamethasone 16mg/d.) can give relief.
- Consider referral for radiotherapy or endoscopic insertion of a stent if appropriate.

*If a terminal event:* Sedate with high doses of midazolam (10–40mg s/cut or slow IV, repeated prn).

**Cough:** Troublesome symptom. Prolonged bouts of coughing are exhausting and frightening – especially if associated with breathlessness and/or haemoptysis.

**Reversible causes:** Box 5.7

**Management:**
*General measures:*
- Exclude any treatable cause for cough (e.g. ACE inhibitors).
- Advise upright body position.
- Steam inhalations, inhalations with menthol or tinct. Benz. Co (Friars balsam) or nebulized saline can help.
- Refer for chest physiotherapy, relaxation and breathing control exercises if tolerated.
- Simple linctus 5–10ml prn can be helpful for dry cough. If not, consider low dose opioid e.g. pholcodine 10mls tds, codeine linctus 30mg qds, Oramorph® 2.5–5mg every 4h. or diamorphine 5–10mg/24h. via syringe driver. If already on opioids ↑ dose by 25%. Titrate dose until symptoms are controlled or side effects.
- Diazepam 2–10mg tds can both relieve anxiety and act as a central cough depressant.

*Specific measures:*
- *Chest infection* – treat with nebulized saline to make secretions less viscous ± antibiotics (if not considered a terminal event).
- *Tumour* – consider referral for radiotherapy.
- *Post-nasal drip* – steam inhalations, steroid nasal spray or drops ± antibiotics.
- *Laryngeal irritation* – try inhaled steroids e.g. beclometasone 100mcgm/actuation 2 puffs bd
- *Bronchospasm* – try bronchodilators ± inhaled or oral steroids
  ⓘ salbutamol may help cough even in the absence of wheeze.
- *Gastric reflux* – try antacids containing dimeticone (Gaviscon®, Asilone®)
- *Lung cancer* – try inhaled sodium cromoglycate 10mg qds; local anaesthesia using nebulized bupivacaine or lidocaine can be helpful – refer for specialist advice (avoid eating/drinking for 1h. afterwards to avoid aspiration). Palliative radiotherapy or chemotherapy can also relieve cough in patients with lung cancer – refer.
- Excess *secretions* – try hyoscine 400–600mcgm 4–8-hourly (or 0.6–2.4mg/24h. via syringe driver) and/or ipratropium inhalers/nebulized ipratropium.

## Box 5.7 Reversible causes of cough

- Infection
- Bronchospasm
- Gastro-oesophageal reflux
- Aspiration
- Drug-induced e.g. ACE inhibitors
- Treatment related e.g. total body irradiation
- Malignant bronchial obstruction/lung metastases
- Heart failure
- Secretions
- Pharyngeal candidiasis

**Further information:**

**Doyle** *et al. Oxford Textbook of Palliative Medicine* (2005). OUP ISBN: 0198566980.

# Haemoptysis

Expectoration of blood or blood-stained sputum.

**Causes:** Box 5.8. Bleeding due to cancer is most commonly from a primary carcinoma of the bronchus and a massive haemoptysis is usually from a squamous cell lung tumour lying centrally or causing cavitation.

## Presentation:
- Small episodes of haemoptysis occasionally herald a catastrophic bleed.
- Malaena rarely occurs in association with haemoptysis if enough blood is swallowed.
- Massive haemoptysis is rare but exceedingly distressing if it occurs.
- The patient is more likely to die from suffocation secondary to the bleed than from the bleed itself.

## Management:

> **Severe, life-threatening bleed:** Make a decision whether the cause of the bleed is treatable or a terminal event. This is best done in advance but bleeding cannot always be predicted.
>
> - **Severe bleed – active treatment:** Briefly assess the severity of the bleed from history and examination. If a significant bleed is suspected:
>   - Call for emergency ambulance support.
>   - Protect the airway
>   - Lie the patient flat and lift their legs higher than body (e.g. feet on pillow). Alternatively, if the side of the bleed is known, lie the patient on that side to protect the healthy lung.
>   - Insert a large bore IV cannula – the opportunity may be lost by the time the ambulance crew arrive. If possible, take a sample for FBC and X-match on insertion.
>   - If available, give oxygen.
>   - If available, start plasma expander/IV fluids.
>   - Transfer as rapidly as possible to hospital.
> - **Severe bleed – no active treatment:**
>   - Stay with the patient.
>   - Give sedative medication e.g. midazolam 20–40mg s/cut or slow IV or diazepam 10–20mg pr, and diamorphine 5–10mg s/cut or IV if in pain.
>   - Support carers as major bleeds are extremely distressing.

*Non-life threatening bleed:* Reassure; monitor frequently.

*Follow up treatment:* Follow up is directed at cause if appropriate:
- Check FBC and clotting screen – if frequent bleeds or large bleed, on anticoagulants or possible bleeding tendency. Consider addressing the clotting problem and/or iron supplements or transfusion (📖 p.106).
- Treat infection that might exacerbate a bleed.
- Consider minimizing bleeding tendency with tranexamic acid 1g tds po – stop if no effect after 1wk. If effective, continue for 1wk. after bleeding has stopped. Continue 500mg tds long-term if bleeding recurs and responds to a further course of treatment. Weigh up benefits of stopping bleeding against ↑ risk of stroke or MI.

- Radiotherapy – consider referral if haemoptysis but not if multiple lung metastases.
- Referral for chemotherapy or palliative surgery e.g. cautery – options in some cases.

### Box 5.8 Causes of haemoptysis

**Respiratory:**
- Lung cancer
- PE (blood is not mixed with sputum)
- TB
- Bronchitis
- Bronchiectasis
- Lung abscess
- Pneumonia
- Violent coughing
- Inhaled foreign body
- Aspergilloma
- Trauma

**Cardiovascular:**
- Mitral stenosis
- Acute LVF

**Other:**
- Collagen vascular disease (e.g. polyarteritis nodosa)
- Bleeding diathesis

### GP Notes:

ⓘ In all patients likely to bleed, consider pre-warning carers and giving them a strategy. Risks of frightening a family with information about possible catastrophic haemoptysis need to be balanced against potential distress that could be caused by leaving a patient and family unprepared – but, can anybody ever be prepared for catastrophic haemoptysis?

# Breathlessness

*'Breathing is the greatest pleasure in life'*
Giovanni Papini (1881–1956)

Breathlessness affects 70% of terminally ill patients. It is usually multifactorial. Breathlessness always has a psychological element – being short of breath is frightening.

**Causes:** Figure 5.5

🛈 If patient has a tracheostomy make sure the tracheostomy tube is not blocked by secretions.

## General management:

### Non-drug measures:
- General reassurance.
- Explanation of reasons for breathlessness and adaptations to lifestyle that might help.
- Proper positioning – improved by sitting upright and straight.
- Try a stream of air over the face – e.g. fan, open window.
- Breathing exercises can help – refer to physiotherapy. Exercises include diaphragmatic breathing and control of breathing rate; relaxation training/distraction training.

### Drug treatment:
- Tenacious secretions – try nebulized saline.
- Oral or subcutaneous opioids ↓ subjective sensation of breathlessness – start with 2.5mg Oramorph® 4 hrly and titrate upwards.
- Try benzodiazepines – 2–5mg diazepam od/bd for background control and lorazepam 1–2mg sublingually prn in between.
- Oxygen has a variable effect and is worth a try.

## Specific measures:
- ***Airway compression, bronchoconstriction or lymphangitis*** – consider referral for anticancer treatment. Otherwise try steroids (dexamethasone 4–8mg/d.).
- ***Intrinsic or extrinsic compression*** – consider referral for radiotherapy, laser therapy or stenting.
- ***Pleural effusion*** – consider referral for drainage ± pleuradesis.
- ***Pericardial effusion*** – consider referral for aspiration in a cardiac unit.
- ***Infection*** – antibiotics ± physiotherapy – have a low threshold so treat with a broad-spectrum antibiotic if appropriate.
- ***Pneumothorax on CXR*** – consider referral for chest drain.
- ***Ascites*** – consider referral for paracentesis if causing breathlessness.
- ***Suspected pulmonary emboli*** – consider anticoagulation (📖 p.154).
- ***Wheeze*** – try inhaled bronchodilators e.g. salbutamol inhaler.
- ***Excessive upper airway secretions*** – try hyoscine 0.4–2.4mg/24h. or glycopyrronium 200–600mcgm/24h. (consult local palliative care team).
- ***Musculoskeletal pain*** – can cause hypoventilation – treat with analgesia.
- ***Anaemia (Hb <9g/l)*** – consider referral for transfusion (📖 p.106).
- ***Thick secretions*** – consider referral for chest physiotherapy.
- ***Vocal cord palsy*** – consider referral to ENT for teflon injection.

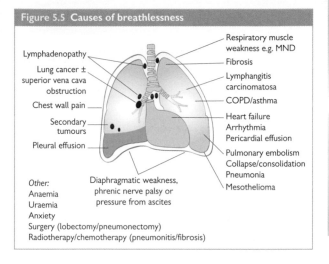

Figure 5.5 Causes of breathlessness

Lymphadenopathy

Lung cancer ± superior vena cava obstruction

Chest wall pain

Secondary tumours

Pleural effusion

Respiratory muscle weakness e.g. MND

Fibrosis

Lymphangitis carcinomatosa

COPD/asthma

Heart failure
Arrhythmia
Pericardial effusion

Pulmonary embolism
Collapse/consolidation
Pneumonia
Mesothelioma

Diaphragmatic weakness, phrenic nerve palsy or pressure from ascites

Other:
Anaemia
Uraemia
Anxiety
Surgery (lobectomy/pneumonectomy)
Radiotherapy/chemotherapy (pneumonitis/fibrosis)

**Superior vena cava obstruction:** 📖 p.152

**Pulmonary embolus:** 📖 p.152

**Breathlessness in motor neurone disease:** 📖 p.177

**Further information:**

Doyle *et al.* Oxford Textbook of Palliative Medicine (2005) OUP. ISBN: 0198566980.

# Hypercalcaemia

Presence of ↑ corrected level of serum calcium (>2.6mmol/l).

**Causes:**
**Common:**
- Malignancy – 10% tumours:
  - Myeloma (>30%)
  - Breast cancer (40%)
  - Other tumours that metastasize to bone – lung, kidney, thyroid, prostate, ovary, colon
  - Squamous cell tumours
- Primary hyperparathyroidism
- Chronic renal failure

**Uncommon:**
- Familial benign hypercalcaemia
- Sarcoidosis
- Thyrotoxicosis
- Milk alkali syndrome
- Vitamin D treatment

**Presentation:** May be an incidental finding. Symptoms are non-specific *'bones, stones, groans and abdominal moans'*
- Tiredness, weakness, and lethargy
- Mild aches and pains
- Thirst, polydipsia, and polyuria
- ↓ appetite, nausea and vomiting
- Abdominal pain
- Constipation
- Depression and/or confusion
- Stone formation or corneal calcification

> ⚠ Always suspect hypercalcaemia if someone is more ill than expected and there is no obvious reason. Untreated hypercalcaemia can be fatal.

**Management:** Depending on the general state of the patient, make a decision whether to treat the hypercalcaemia or not.

**If a decision is made not to treat:** provide symptom control and don't check the serum calcium again.

**Active treatment:** depends on level of symptoms and $Ca^{2+}$:
- *Asymptomatic patient with corrected calcium <3mmol/l:* Monitor.
- *Symptomatic and/or corrected calcium >3mmol/l:*
  - Arrange treatment with IV fluids and bisphosphonates via oncologist/palliative care team immediately.
  - Check serum calcium 7–10d. post-treatment. 20% of patients do not respond and there is no benefit retreating them.
  - Effect of bisphosphonate lasts 20–30d.. Consider maintenance with oral bisphosphonates started 1wk. after the initial IV treatment or regular IV bisphosphonate. Many initially responsive to bisphosphonates become unresponsive with time.

## GP Notes: Checking $Ca^{2+}$

Check calcium level on an *uncuffed* sample to avoid falsely high readings.

Correct for serum albumin – for every mmol/l less than 40, a correction of 0.02mmol/l should be added to the serum calcium concentration measured. *For example:*

$Ca^{2+}$    2.40      Corrected $Ca^{2+}$ = $(40 - 24) \times 0.02 + 2.4$
Albumin   24                   = $0.32 + 2.4$ = **2.72**

# Diabetes in palliative care

Fine control of blood glucose levels is no longer appropriate in the last weeks of illness – it may not be possible and is a distracting burden for the patient and family. Treatment goal is to keep the patient asymptomatic from their DM (avoiding symptomatic hyperglycaemia and hypoglycaemia) and to ↓ the burden of care (e.g. stop inappropriate glucose monitoring).

## Causes of hyperglycaemia in palliative care:

- Pre-existing DM – treatment needs may change e.g. if started on high-calorie feeds or corticosteroids, or if the patient develops infection.
- Corticosteroid-induced DM – dose-related effect. Ask patients on long-term steroids to check their urine for glucose weekly.
- Insulin deficiency due to pancreatic cancer.

## Unpleasant symptoms caused by hyperglycaemia:

- Persisting or frequent infection
- Thirst
- Polyuria
- Nausea and vomiting
- Blurred vision and/or neurological symptoms
- Confusion
- Ketoacidosis/coma

## Causes of hypoglycaemia in palliative care:

- ↓ appetite and/or cachexia.
- Nausea or vomiting – due to cancer or treatment (e.g. chemotherapy).
- Liver replacement by tumour – results in low glycogen stores and limited gluconeogenesis.
- Excess hypoglycaemic agents – treatment needs for DM change e.g. if a patient loses a lot of weight, s/he may need less oral hypoglycaemic agent or insulin to control blood sugars.
- Insulin-secreting tumours—rare.

## Management:

- **Diet-controlled type 2 DM** – none. Only monitor if symptomatic.
- **Oral hypoglycaemic-controlled type 2 DM** – Use short-acting hypoglycaemic agents e.g. gliclazide. ↓ drug dose aiming to stop drugs. Stop drugs if unable to eat or drink. Check BM 1–2x/wk. routinely and if any symptoms of hypo- or hyperglycaemia.
- **Insulin-controlled type 2 DM** – ↓ dose of insulin, aiming to stop insulin if possible. Check BM daily. If BM >20mmol/l or symptomatic, restart insulin in as simple a regime as possible (see type 1 DM). If symptoms then improve and there are no BMs <4mmol/l after 2d. of monitoring, stop monitoring unless symptomatic hypo- or hyperglycaemia. Stop insulin if unable to eat or drink.
- **Insulin dependent type 1 DM** – continue as simple an insulin regime as possible (e.g. human monotard od, insulin glargine od or human isophane insulin ²/₃ daily dose man and ¹/₃ nocte), checking BM prior to giving insulin. Aim to keep blood sugar at 10–15mmol/l. The priority is to prevent hypoglycaemia. Continue insulin even if not eating.

## Initiating treatment in new diagnosis of hyperglycaemia:

**Blood glucose ↑ but asymptomatic:**

- Give dietary advice tailored to individual circumstances.
- Consider infection as a cause. Treat any infection found.
- If on corticosteroids, consider reducing dose or stopping.

**Blood glucose ↑ and symptomatic:** Check urine for ketones. If ketones present or blood glucose >27mmol/L, consider admission or same day referral for specialist advice on treatment, depending on the clinical state of the patient.

*If no ketones and BM <27:*

- Give dietary advice tailored to circumstances.
- Exclude infection as a cause. Treat any infection found.
- If on corticosteroids, consider reducing dose or stopping.
- If BM is still high and patient is symptomatic, start an oral hypoglycaemic agent e.g. gliclazide 80mg od.
- Thin, cachectic patients are less likely to respond to oral hypoglycaemic drugs. If not responding, consider switching to insulin early – take specialist advice.

### GP Notes: Converting insulin

If converting from a mixed insulin regime (e.g. isophane insulin + human soluble insulin) to single daily human monotard:

1. Calculate the total daily insulin requirement
2. Reduce the dose by 20–30%
3. Give this dose once daily as human monotard (usually at night)
4. Check BMs pre-dose and if symptomatic
5. Adjust the dose as necessary

## Further information:

**Palliative Medicine** Boyd K Diabetes mellitus in hospice patients: some guidelines (1993) **7** p.163–4.

# Neurological and orthopaedic problems

**Dysarthria:** Difficulty with articulation due to inco-ordination or weakness of the musculature of speech. Language is normal. Ask to repeat 'baby hippopotamus' or 'British constitution'. Treat the cause if possible otherwise, support with speech therapy and aids to communication.

*Causes:*
- *Cerebellar disease* – slurring as if drunk. Speech is irregular in volume and scanning in quality.
- *Extrapyramidal disease* e.g. Parkinson's disease – soft, indistinct, and monotonous.
- *Pseudo-bulbar palsy* – Patients may present with alteration of speech – typically nasal speech sounding like Donald Duck, difficulty swallowing or chewing. The tongue is spastic and jaw jerk ↑. *Causes:* stroke (bilateral); MS; MND.
- *Bulbar palsy* – Loss of function of the tongue, muscles of chewing/ swallowing ± facial muscles. *Examination:* flaccid, fasciculating tongue, jaw jerk normal or absent, speech – quiet, hoarse, or nasal. *Causes:* MND, Guillain-Barré syndrome, alcoholic brain stem myelinolysis (central pontine myelinolysis), brain stem tumours (1° or 2°), syringobulbia, polio, hyponatraemia.

**Management:**
- Treat reversible causes if possible.
- Involve the speech therapist early to teach the patient techniques relevant to their own special needs.
- Various aids to communication are available e.g. lightwriters with or without synthesized voice function. Other computerized systems are available from specialized centres including electronic equipment, telephone devices and communication boards which may be adapted to the physical abilities of the individual patient.

🛈 It is essential to plan ahead – motor function may deteriorate rapidly.

**Raised intracranial pressure:** Occurs with 1° or 2° brain tumours.
*Features:* Characterized by:
- Headache – worse on lying
- Vomiting
- Confusion
- Diplopia
- Convulsions
- Papilloedema

**Management:**
- Unless a terminal event, refer patients urgently to neurosurgery for assessment. Options include insertion of a shunt or cranial radiotherapy.
- If no further active treatment is appropriate, start symptomatic treatment – raise the head of the bed, start dexamethasone 16mg/d. (stop if no response in 1wk.), provide analgesia.

**Generalized myoclonic twitching:** May occur during the terminal stages of illness and if uraemic. Treat with anticonvulsants (e.g. sodium valproate 300mg bd) if able to manage oral medication. If unable to manage oral medication treat with clonazepam 1–4mg/24h. s/cut, midazolam 20–100mg/24h. s/cut or phenobarbital 200–600mg/24h. s/cut.

**Spinal cord compression:** Affects 5% of cancer patients – 70% in the thoracic region. Presentation can be subtle. Maintain a *high* level of suspicion in all cancer patients who complain of back pain – especially those with known bony metastases or tumours likely to metastasize to bone.

**Presentation:**
- Often back pain, worse on movement, appears before neurology.
- Neurological symptoms/signs can be non-specific – constipation, weak legs, urinary hesitancy.
- Lesions above L1 (lower end of spinal cord) may produce UMN signs (e.g. ↑ tone & reflexes) and a sensory level.
- Lesions below L1 may produce LMN signs (↓ tone & reflexes) and peri-anal numbness (cauda equina syndrome).

**Management:** Prompt treatment (<24–48h. from 1ˢᵗ neurological symptoms) is needed if there is any hope of restoring function. Once paralysed, <5% walk again. Treat with oral dexamethasone 16mg/d. and refer urgently for assessment and surgery/radiotherapy unless in final stages of disease.

**Bone fractures:** Common in advanced cancer due to osteoporosis, trauma as a result of falls, or metastases. Have a low index of suspicion if a new bony pain develops.

⚠ In the elderly, fracture of a long bone can present as acute confusion.

**Management:**
- Analgesia
- Unless in a very terminal state, confirm the fracture on x-ray and refer to orthopaedics or radiotherapy urgently for consideration of fixation (long bones, wrist, neck of femur) and/or radiotherapy (rib fractures, vertebral fractures).

# Venous thromboembolism

### Risk factors for venous thromboembolism:
- Malignancy (~50%–10% have symptoms)
- Age >40y.
- Smoking
- Obesity
- Immobility
- Recent long distance travel
- Recent trauma and/or surgery
- COC pill/HRT use
- Heart failure
- Nephrotic syndrome
- Inflammatory bowel disease
- PMH of thromboembolism
- Inherited clotting disorder

**Deep vein thrombosis (DVT):** Any deep vein can clot. Common sites are the limbs, mesentery, cerebral sinus, and retina. DVT in the leg (commonest site) may be proximal – involving veins above the knee – or isolated to the calf veins.

**Presentation:** Unilateral leg pain, swelling and/or tenderness ± mild fever, pitting oedema, warmth and distended collateral superficial veins.

### Differential diagnosis:
- Cellulitis
- Haematoma
- Ruptured Baker's cyst
- Superficial thrombophlebitis
- Chronic venous insufficiency
- Venous obstruction
- Post-thrombotic syndrome
- Acute arterial ischaemia
- Lymphoedema
- Fracture
- Hypoproteinaemia

**Investigation:** Clinical diagnosis is unreliable.
- Only 50% of DVTs are symptomatic.
- <50% with clinically suspected DVT have diagnosis confirmed on diagnostic imaging.

The relevance of active management of DVT in patients with advanced disease will depend on the stage of disease and symptoms. If active management is appropriate, refer for further assessment. Many hospitals have rapid access facilities for diagnosis, bypassing conventional admission.

*Specialist assessment:* All patients with malignancy fall into a high-risk group and require USS. If USS is positive, diagnosis of DVT is confirmed.

If USS is negative, USS is repeated after 1wk. or the patient is assessed with venography, CT or MRI.

### Active management of patients with confirmed DVT:
- Initial anticoagulation is with low molecular weight heparin (LMWH) followed by oral anticoagulation (warfarin) – usually as an outpatient.
- LMWH should be continued for at least 4d. and until the INR is in the therapeutic range for ≥2d.. Target INR is 2.5 (range 2–3).
- Oral anticoagulants ↓ risk of further thromboembolism and should be continued until no longer appropriate in patients with terminal illness.
- Graduated elastic compression stockings – ↓ risk post-thrombotic leg syndrome by 12–50%.

## GP Notes: Anticoagulation without confirmation of diagnosis

It is not uncommon for terminally ill patients to be distressed by:
- Leg/torso oedema – possible inferior vena cava thrombosis.
- Acute/increasing breathlessness – possible PE.

In these situations, if there is a high suspicion of venous thromboembolism, it may be justifiable to start anticoagulation before formal diagnosis if the patient is not fit enough for investigation or declines admission. Treatment (particularly for PE) may improve symptoms significantly in <48h. Discuss with palliative care team.

## Advice for patients: Information and support for patients

**Lifeblood: The Thrombosis Charity** ☎ 0207 633 9937
🖥 www.thrombosis-charity.org.uk

**Pulmonary embolus (PE):** Venous thrombi – usually from a DVT – pass into the pulmonary circulation and block blood flow to the lungs.

**Presentation:**
- *Symptoms:* Acute dyspnoea, pleuritic chest pain, haemoptysis, syncope.
- *Signs:*
  - Hypotension
  - Tachycardia
  - Cyanosis
  - Tachypnoea
  - Pleural rub
  - ↑ JVP
- Look for a source of emboli – often DVT is not clinically obvious.

⚠ Have a high level of suspicion. Patients may have minimal symptoms/signs apart from some pleuritis pain and dyspnoea.

**Differential diagnosis:**
- Pneumonia and pleurisy.
- MI/unstable angina.
- Other causes of acute breathlessness – acute LVF, asthma, exacerbation of COPD, pneumothorax, shock (e.g. due to anaphylaxis), arrhythmia, hyperventilation.
- Other causes of acute chest pain – aortic dissection, rib fracture, musculoskeletal chest pain, pericarditis, oesophageal spasm, shingles.

**Management:** Make a decision whether active management is appropriate. PE may be the terminal event.

*Active management:* If suspected, give oxygen as soon as possible and admit as an acute medical emergency. Specialist management involves investigation to prove diagnosis (Ventilation-perfusion (VQ) scan, MRI and/or pulmonary angiography). Thrombolytic therapy is controversial. In all cases of proven PE, anticoagulation is started. In terminally ill patients, warfarin should be continued until no longer appropriate, aiming to keep the INR ≈2.5 (range 2–3).

**Superior vena cava (SVC) obstruction:** Due to infiltration of the vessel wall, clot within the superior vena cava or extrinsic pressure. 75% are due to 1° lung cancer. Lymphoma is the other major cause (15%).

**Presentation:**
- Shortness of breath/stridor.
- Headache worse on stooping ± visual disturbance ± dizziness/ collapse.
- Swelling of the face – particularly around the eyes, neck, hands and arms, and/or injected cornea.
- *Examination:* look for non-pulsatile distention of neck veins and dilated collateral veins (seen as small dilated veins over the anterior chest wall below the clavicles) in which blood courses downwards.

**Management:**
- Treat breathlessness (sit patient upright and give 60% oxygen).
- Treat pain/panic with opioids – 5mg Oramorph® 4 hourly ± benzodiazepine depending on the level of anxiety.
- Start corticosteroid (dexamethasone 16mg/d.).
- Refer urgently for oncology opinion. Palliative radiotherapy has a response rate of 70%. Stenting ± thrombolysis is also an option.

# Anticoagulation in palliative care

Rapid changes in clinical state, liver involvement, drug interactions and difficulties of monitoring make anticoagulation difficult in patients with advanced disease.

**Heparin in the community:** Only use on specialist advice. Usually s/cut low molecular weight heparin (LMWH) is used as it does not need daily monitoring.

## Warfarin:

- Patients with cancer taking warfarin have a higher incidence of bleeding than those without cancer.
- If the patient develops recurrent thrombosis, warfarin is less effective than heparin – discuss transferring to heparin with the local palliative care team or consultant in charge of the patient's care.
- Patients on warfarin (for whatever reason) who have cancer and in whom the INR is hard to control, may benefit from being switched to LMWH – discuss with palliative care team or consultant in charge of the patient's care.

**Monitoring warfarin:** Table 5.11. If there is a change in clinical state monitor more frequently until steady state is re-established. Have an explicit system for handling results promptly, making informed decisions on further treatment and testing, and communicating results to patients. Monitor the process with regular audit.

**Terminal situation:** If the patient is clearly in the terminal stage, both warfarin and LMWH can be stopped.

| Table 5.11 Warfarin therapy: Recall periods during maintenance therapy | |
|---|---|
| **INR** | **Recall interval and action** |
| 1 INR high<br>⚠ If INR > 8 – admit | ↑ risk of bleeding. Stop treatment for 1–3d. (max 1wk. in prosthetic valve patients) and restart at a lower dose. Recall 7–14d. |
| 1 INR low | ↑ risk of thromboembolism. ↑ dose and recall in 7–14d. |
| 1 therapeutic INR | Recall 4wk. |
| 2 therapeutic INRs | Recall 6wk. (maximum interval if prosthetic heart valve) |
| 3 therapeutic INRs | Recall 8wk.* |
| 4 therapeutic INRs | Recall 10wk.* |
| 5 therapeutic INRs | Recall 12wk.* |
| * Except prosthetic heart valves where maximum recall interval is 6wk. | |

## GMS Contract

Anticoagulation monitoring may be provided by practices as a national enhanced service (📖 p.267).

## Table 5.12 Indications for oral anticoagulation and target INR

| Indication | Target INR (target range) | Duration of treatment |
|---|---|---|
| *Cardiac:* | | |
| Mechanical prosthetic heart valves: | | |
| 1st generation | 3.5 (3.0–4.0) | Long term |
| 2nd second generation | 3.0 (2.5–3.5) | Long term |
| Rheumatic mitral valve disease | 2.5 (2.0–3.0) | Long term |
| Valvular AF and AF due to congenital heart disease or thyrotoxicosis | 2.5 (2.0–3.0) | Long term |
| Non-valvular AF and medium/high risk of stroke | 2.5 (2.0–3.0) | Long term |
| Dilated cardiomyopathy | 2.5 (2.0–3.0) | Long term |
| Mural thrombus post MI | 2.5 (2.0–3.0) | 3mo. |
| Cardioversion | 2.5 (2.0–3.0) | 3wk. before procedure and for 4wk. after procedure |
| *Venous thromboembolism:* | | |
| 1st PE/DVT and persistent risk factors e.g. cancer, immobility | 2.5 (2.0–3.0) | Long term |
| Prophylaxis of recurrent DVT/PE | | |
|   occurring on warfarin | 3.5 (3.0–4.0) | Long term |
|   occurring off warfarin | 2.5 (2.0–3.0) | Long term |
| *Other disorders:* | | |
| Inherited thrombophilia with no previous thrombosis | 2.5 (2.0–3.0) | Anticoagulate for high-risk activities e.g. surgery |
| Inherited thrombophilia with previous episode of thrombosis | 2.5 (2.0–3.0) | Long term |
| Antiphospholipid syndrome | 2.5–3.5 | Long term |

⚠ Warfarin can be a dangerous drug:
- It causes numerous admissions every year with bleeding.
- It interacts with a large number of drugs, including aspirin, some antibiotics, cimetidine, corticosteroids, and NSAIDs.

### Further information:
SIGN Antithrombotic therapy (1999) ⌨ www.sign.ac.uk
British Journal of Haematology Guidelines on oral anticoagulation (3rd edition – 1999) **101**: 374–87. ⌨ www.bcshguidelines.com

# Lymphoedema

Lymphoedema is due to obstruction of lymphatic drainage resulting in oedema with high protein content. It usually affects a limb but may affect more than one limb, the head, trunk, or genitals.

## Risk factors:

- ♀ > ♂
- ↑ with age
- Obesity
- Lack of physical exercise

## Causes:

- Axillary, groin, or intrapelvic tumour.
- Treatment of tumour – axillary or groin surgery, postoperative infection, or radiotherapy.
- Rarely primary (congenital abnormality of lymph tissue) or secondary to DVT, trauma, infection, or inflammatory arthritis.

## Presentation:

- Swollen limb ± pitting
- Impaired limb mobility and function
- Discomfort/pain related to tissue swelling and/or shoulder strain
- Neuralgia pain – especially when axillary nodes are involved
- Psychological distress

**Management:** Untreated lymphoedema becomes increasingly resistant to treatment due to chronic inflammation and subcutaneous fibrosis.

**Avoid injury:** In at-risk patients (e.g. patients who have had breast cancer with axillary clearance) or those with lymphoedema, injury to the limb may precipitate or worsen lymphoedema. Avoid sunburn and cuts (e.g. wear gloves for gardening). Do not take blood from the limb or use the limb for IV access, vaccination or BP measurement.

### Skin hygiene:

- Keep the skin in good condition with moisturisers e.g. aqueous cream.
- Treat fungal infections with topical agents e.g. clotrimazole cream.
- Cellulitis is a common complication and causes rapid ↑ in swelling. Treat with oral antibiotics (e.g. penicillin V 500mg qds). If ≥2 episodes of cellulitis consider prophylactic antibiotics e.g. penicillin V 250mg bd.

### External support:

- Intensive support can be provided with compression bandages – refer to specialist physiotherapy or the palliative care team.
- Maintenance therapy with a lymphoedema sleeve is helpful – contact the palliative care team or breast care specialist nurse for information.

**Exercise:** Advise gentle daily exercise of the affected limb, gradually increasing range of movement. 🛈 Patients should wear compression bandages or a lymphoedema sleeve whilst doing their exercises.

**Massage:** Very gentle finger tip massage in the line of drainage of the lymphatics can help – refer to specialist physiotherapist for advice.

**Diuretics:** If the condition develops/deteriorates after corticosteroid or NSAID use, or if there is a venous component, consider trial of diuretics e.g furosemide 20mg od. Otherwise, diuretics are of no benefit.

## Figure 5.6 Lymphoedema of the right arm

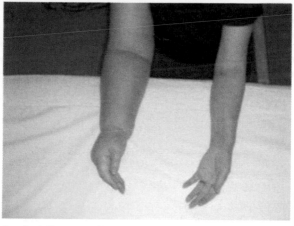

Reproduced with permission of Harlington Hospice 🖳 www.harlingtonhospice.org

---

**Advice for patients: Information and support for patients and carers**

Lymphoedema Support Network ☎ 020 7351 0990
🖳 www.lymphoedema.org/lsn
UKLymph.com Online support network 🖳 www.uklymph.com

**Information leaflets on lymphoedema:**
Skin Care Campaign 🖳 www.skincarecampaign.org
CancerHelp UK 🖳 www.cancerhelp.org.uk
Royal Marsden Hospital 🖳 www.royalmarsden.org.uk
Vascular Society 🖳 www.vascularsociety.org.uk/

**Further information:**
**Cochrane** Badger et al.. *Physical therapies for reducing and controlling lymphoedema of the limb* (2004).

# Wound care

**Bed sores:**
- Due to pressure necrosis of the skin.
- Immobile patients are at high risk – especially if frail ± incontinent.
- Likely sites of pressure damage – shoulder blades, elbows, spine, buttocks, knees, ankles, and heels.
- Bed sores heal slowly in terminally ill patients and are a source of discomfort and stress for both patients and carers (who often feel guilty that a pressure sore is a mark of poor care).
- If at risk refer to the DN for palliative care nursing team for advice on prevention of bed sores – protective mattresses and cushions, incontinence advice, advice on positioning and movement.
- Warn carers to make contact with the DN or palliative care nursing team if a red patch does not improve 24h. after relieving the pressure on the area.
- Treat aggressively any sores that develop and admit if not resolving.

**Wound care:**
- Large wounds can have major impact on quality of life.
- Patients with advanced disease have major risk factors for development and poor healing of wounds – immobility, poor nutrition, skin infiltration ± breakdown due to malignancy.
- Skin infiltration causing ulceration or fungating wounds can be particularly distressing.

**Management:** The primary aim is comfort. Healing is a secondary aim and may be impossible. Always involve the DN and/or specialist palliative care nursing team early. Many hospitals also have wound care specialist nurses who are invaluable sources of advice.

**Specific management problems:** Table 5.13

**Body image:** Odour, obvious dressings, facial disfigurement and asymmetry can result in altered body image. As a result, patients may become socially isolated and experience difficulties in their relationships with their relatives/friends – including sexual problems.

**Management:**
- Talk to the patient and carers – give information and explanation.
- Empathetic listening is often therapeutic in itself.
- Ensure dressings are as leakproof and/or odourproof as possible.
- Tailor dressings to the patient's needs e.g. if going to a social event, avoid bulky or unsightly dressings.
- Consider counselling and/or management of depression or anxiety associated with altered body image, where necessary.

**Methicillin-resistant Staphylococcus aureus (MRSA):** Is difficult to eradicate. If causing the patient problems, discuss management with the local microbiology team. In all cases, warn health care professionals in contact with the patient and any health or social care establishment the patient will visit that the patient is MRSA+ve so that appropriate precautions can be taken to prevent spread to other patients.

## Table 5.13 Common wound management problems

| Problem | Management |
|---------|------------|
| Pain | Exclude infection.<br>Ensure the dressing is comfortable.<br>Limit frequency of dressing changes.<br>Ensure adequate background analgesia.<br>Consider additional analgesia if needed for dressing changes and/or topical opioids on the dressing. |
| Excessive exudate | Use high-absorbency dressings with further packing on top ± plastic pads to protect clothing.<br>Change the top layer of the dressing as often as needed but avoid frequent changes of the dressing placed directly on the wound.<br>Protect the surrounding skin with a barrier cream/spray. |
| Necrotic tissue | Use desloughing agents.<br>Referral for surgical debridement may be necessary. |
| Bleeding | Prevent bleeding during dressing changes by:<br>• Avoiding frequent dressing changes.<br>• Using non-adherent dressings or dressings which liquefy and can be washed off (e.g. Sorbsan®).<br>• Irrigating the wound with saline to remove dressings.<br>If there is surface bleeding – put pressure on the wound; if pressure is not working try:<br>• Kaltostat®<br>• Adrenaline – 1mg/ml or 1:1000 on a gauze pad.<br>• Sucralfate liquid – place on a non-adherent dressing and apply firmly to the bleeding area.<br>Consider referral for radiotherapy or palliative surgery (e.g. cautery). |
| Odour | Treat with systemic and/or topical metronidazole.<br>Charcoal dressings can be helpful.<br>Seal the wound e.g. with additional layer of clingfilm dressing.<br>Try disguising the smell with deodorisers (e.g. Nilodor®) used sparingly on top of the dressing – short-term measure. Long-term, the deodorant smell often becomes associated with the smell of the wound for the patient. |
| Infection | Usually chronic and localized.<br>Irrigate the wound with warm saline or under running water in the shower/bath.<br>If the surrounding skin is inflamed, swab the wound and send for M, C&S then start oral antibiotics e.g. flucloxacillin 250–500mg qds or erythromycin 250–500mg qds.<br>Alter antibiotics depending on sensitivities of the organisms grown. |

159

## Further information:

**Tissue Viability Society** Information on bed sores ⊟ www.tvs.org.uk
**NICE** Pressure ulcer management (2005) ⊟ www.nice.org.uk

# Insomnia

From the Latin meaning 'no sleep'. Describes a perception of disturbed or inadequate sleep. Affects ~1:4 of the UK population (♀>♂), thought to suffer in varying degrees. Prevalence ↑ with age, rising to 1:2 amongst the over 65s. Causes are numerous – common examples include:

* *Minor, self-limiting:* travel, stress, shift work, small children, arousal.
* *Psychological:* >½ have mental health problems – depression, anxiety, mania, grief, alcoholism.
* *Physical:* drugs (e.g. steroids), pain, nausea or vomiting, pruritus, tinnitus, sweats, nocturia, breathlessness, restless legs.

## Definition of 'a good night's sleep':

* <30 min. to fall asleep
* Maintenance of sleep for 6–8h.
* <3 brief awakenings/night
* Feeling well rested and refreshed on awakening.

**Management:** Careful evaluation. Many patients do not have a sleep problem themselves but a relative feels there is a problem e.g. the retired milkman continuing to wake at 4a.m.. Others have unrealistic expectations e.g. they need 12h. sleep/d.. Reassurance alone may be all that is required.

### For genuine problems:

* ***Eliminate as far as possible any physical problems preventing sleep*** e.g. treat asthma; give long acting pain killers to last the whole night; treat nausea/vomiting (📖 p.114).
* ***Treat psychiatric problems*** e.g. depression, anxiety.
* ***Sleep hygiene*** – Box 5.9
* ***Relaxation techniques*** – Audiotapes (borrow from libraries or buy from pharmacies); relaxation classes (often offered by local recreation centres/adult education centres/palliative care services); many physiotherapists can teach relaxation techniques.
* ***Consider drug treatment:*** Last resort. Benzodiazepines may be prescribed for insomnia 'only when it is severe, disabling, or subjecting the individual to extreme distress.'

**Drug treatment:** Benzodiazepines (e.g. temazepam), zolpidem, zopiclone and low-dose TCA (e.g. amitriptyline 25–50mg) nocte are all commonly prescribed for patients with insomnia.

* *Side effects:* amnesia and daytime somnolence. Most hypnotics do affect daytime performance and may cause falls in the elderly (use with care and only in low doses). Warn patients about their effect on driving and operating machinery.
* Only prescribe a few weeks' supply at a time due to potential for dependence and abuse.

> ⚠ Don't forget the carer who will often also have fragmented nights but still have to perform caring tasks during the day.

**Complications of insomnia:** ↓ quality of life; ↓ concentration and memory affecting performance of daytime tasks; relationship problems; risk of accidents. 10% of motor accidents are related to tiredness.

---

### Box 5.9 Principles of 'sleep hygiene'

- Don't go to bed until you feel sleepy.
- Don't stay in bed if you are not asleep.
- Avoid daytime naps.
- Establish a regular bedtime routine.
- Reserve a room for sleep only (if possible). Do not eat, read, work or watch TV in it.
- Make sure the bedroom and bed are comfortable, and avoid extremes of noise and temperature.
- Avoid caffeine, alcohol, and nicotine.
- Have a warm bath and warm milky drink at bedtime.
- Take regular exercise but avoid late night hard exercise (sex is OK).
- Monitor your sleep with a sleep diary (record both the times you sleep and its quality).
- Rise at the same time every morning regardless of how long you've slept.

---

### GP Notes: Patients with dementia

- Tend to sleep less deeply and wake more frequently.
- Often need constant reassurance and to sleep in a lit room to minimize disorientation.
- Hypnotics may aggravate the situation by increasing confusion.
- Alternatives include haloperidol 0.5–2mg or risperidone 0.5–1mg – give in the early evening to allow time to act.

🕒 Risperidone should not be used if there is a history of cerebrovascular disease.

---

### Advice for patients: information and support

**Royal College of Psychiatrists.** Patient information sheets
🖥 www.rcpsych.ac.uk

# Acute confusional states (delirium)

Common condition – particularly amongst elderly patients. May occur *de novo* or be superimposed upon chronic confusion of dementia resulting in sudden worsening of cognition.

**Presentation:**
- Global cognitive deficit with onset over hours/days.
- Fluctuating conscious level – typically worse at night/late afternoon.
- Impaired memory – on recovery, amnesia of the events is usual.
- Disorientation in time and place.
- Odd behaviour – may be underactive, drowsy and/or withdrawn *or* hyperactive and agitated.
- Disordered thinking – often slow and muddled ± delusions (e.g. accuse relatives of taking things).
- Disturbed perceptions – hallucinations (particularly visual) are common.
- Mood swings.

**Examination:** Can be difficult. If possible, do a thorough general physical examination to exclude treatable causes.

**Possible causes:** Table 5.14

**Differential diagnosis:**
- *Deafness* – may appear confused.
- *Dementia* – longer history and lack of fluctuations in conscious level – in practice may be difficult to distinguish especially if you come across a patient who is alone and can give no history.
- *Primary mental illness* e.g. schizophrenia; anxiety state; depression.

**Management:** Is aimed at treating all remediable causes.

Admit if:
- The patient lives alone.
- The patient will be left unsupervised for any duration of time.
- If carers (or residential home) are unprepared/unable to continue looking after the patient.
- If history and examination have indicated a cause requiring acute hospital treatment, admit as an emergency – if necessary under a section.

Possible investigations to consider in the community:
- Urine – dipstick for glucose, ketones, blood, protein, nitrates and white cells, send for M, C&S.
- BM to exclude hypoglycaemia.
- Blood – FBC, ESR, U&E, $Ca^{2+}$, LFTs, TFTs.
- ECG.
- CXR.

**Management at home:**

- Acute confusion is frightening for patients and carers – reassure and support them.
- Treat the cause if clinically appropriate e.g. antibiotics for UTI or chest infection.
- Try to avoid sedation as this can make confusion worse. Where unavoidable use haloperidol 1–2mg prn or lorazepam 0.5–1mg prn.
- Involve district or palliative care nursing services e.g. to provide incontinence aids, cot sides, moral support.
- If the cause does not become clear despite investigation, or the patient fails to improve with treatment, and the patient is not near to death, admit for further investigation and assessment.
- If a terminal event – 📖 p.192.

| Table 5.14 Causes of acute confusion | |
|---|---|
| Infection | Particularly UTI, pneumonia; rarely encephalitis, meningitis |
| Drugs | Opiates, sedatives, steroids, L-dopa, anticonvulsants, recreational drugs, digoxin or lithium toxicity |
| Metabolic | Hypoglycaemia, uraemia, liver failure, hyper-calcaemia, other electrolyte imbalance (rarer) |
| Alcohol or drug withdrawal | |
| Hypoxia | e.g. severe pneumonia, exacerbation of COPD, cardiac failure |
| Cardiovascular | MI, stroke, TIA |
| Intracranial | Space-occupying lesion (e.g. cerebral metastasis), raised intracranial pressure, head injury (especially subdural haematoma) |
| Thyroid disease | Hyper- or hypothyroidism |
| Carcinomatosis | |
| Epilepsy | Temporal lobe epilepsy, post-ictal state |
| Pain | |
| Constipation | |
| Urinary retention | |
| Nutritional deficiency | $B_{12}$, thiamine or nicotinic acid deficiency |

# Psychiatric problems

**Anxiety:** All patients with terminal disease are anxious at times for a variety of reasons including fear of uncontrolled symptoms and of being left alone to die. When anxiety starts interfering with quality of life, intervention is justified.

### Management:
*Non-drug measures:* often all that is needed:
- Acknowledgement of the patient's anxiety.
- Full explanation of questions + written information as needed.
- Support – self-help groups, day care, patients groups, specialist home nurses (e.g. Macmillan nurses).
- Relaxation training and training in breathing control.
- Physical therapies e.g. aromatherapy, art therapy, exercise.

*Drug measures:*
- *Acute anxiety:* Try lorazepam 1–2mg sl prn or diazepam 2–10mg prn.
- *Chronic anxiety:* Try an antidepressant e.g. sertraline 50mg od. Alternatives include regular diazepam e.g. 5–10mg od/bd, haloperidol 1–3mg bd/tds or β–blockers e.g. propranolol 40mg od–tds – watch for postural hypotension.

If anxiety is not responding to simple measures, seek specialist help from either the psychiatric or palliative care team.

**Depression:** A terminal diagnosis makes patients sad. 10–20% of terminally ill patients develop clinical depression but, in practice, it is often difficult to decide whether a patient is depressed or just appropriately sad about his/her diagnosis and its implications. Many symptoms of terminal disease (e.g. poor appetite) are also symptoms of depression so screening questionnaires for depression are often unhelpful. If in doubt, a trial of antidepressants can help.

**Assessment of suicide risk:** Ask about suicidal ideas and plans in a sensitive but probing way. It is a common misconception that asking about suicide can plant the idea into a patient's head and make suicide more likely. Evidence is to the contrary.

### Management:
*Non-drug measures:*
- Support e.g. day and/or respite care; carers group; specialist nurse support (e.g. Macmillan nurse; CPN); ↑ help in the home.
- Relaxation – often ↑ the patient's feeling of control over the situation.
- Explanation – of worries/problems/concerns about the future.
- Physical activity – exercise, writing.

*Drug measures:*
- Consider starting an antidepressant – Table 5.15.
- All antidepressants take ~2wk. to work.
- If immediate effect is required, consider using flupentixol 1mg od (beware as can cause psychomotor agitation).

If not responding, or suicidal, refer for psychiatric opinion.

## GP Notes: Assessment of anxiety

*Ask:*
1. Is it severe?
2. Is it long-standing?
3. Is it due to alcohol withdrawal?
4. Is it situational?
5. Is it related to a specific fear?
6. Is the family anxious?

## Table 5.15 Drug treatment of depression *(BNF 4.3)*

| Drug group and examples | Features |
|---|---|
| *Selective serotonin re-uptake inhibitors (SSRIs)* e.g. fluoxetine 20mg od | Usually first choice as less likely to be discontinued due to side effects. Warn of possible anxiety and agitation and advise patients to stop if significant. GI side effects, including dyspepsia, are common. |
| *Tricyclic anti-depressants (TCAs)* e.g. lofepramine 70mg od/bd/tds | Titrate dose up from low dose until the patient feels it is helping, or until side effects intrude. Common side effects include drowsiness, dry mouth, blurred vision, constipation, urinary retention and sweating. |
| *Monoamine oxidase inhibitors (MAOIs)* e.g. phenelzine 15mg tds | MAOIs should not be started until at least 1–2wk. after a tricyclic has been stopped (3wk. in the case of clomipramine or imipramine). Other antidepressants should not be started for 2wk. after treatment with MAOIs has been stopped (3wk. if starting clomipramine or imipramine). |
| *Serotonin and nonadrenaline re-uptake inhibitors (SNRIs)* e.g. venlafaxine 37.5mg bd | Effective antidepressants with side effect profile similar to SSRIs. |
| *St. John's Wort* | May be effective in mild depression but formulations vary widely in potency. Side effects include dry mouth, gastrointestinal symptoms, fatigue, dizziness, skin rashes and ↑ sensitivity to sunlight. Interacts with many drugs including antidepressants (especially SSRIs – sweating, shivering, muscle contractions), anticonvulsants (↓ effects), warfarin, oral contraceptives, ciclosporin, digoxin and theophylline. ⚠ Do not use concurrently with prescription antidepressants; discontinue 2wk. prior to surgery due to theoretical risk of interaction with anaesthetic agents. |

# Chronic obstructive pulmonary disease (COPD)

Slowly progressive disorder characterized by airflow obstruction. COPD is the commonest chronic respiratory disorder requiring palliation. Many symptoms experienced by cancer patients and patients with COPD are similar: cancer patients' symptoms may be more severe, but those of COPD patients tend to be more prolonged.

## History:
- Shortness of breath on exertion – use an objective measure e.g. MRC dyspnoea scale (Table 5.16) to grade breathlessness
- Chronic cough
- Regular sputum production
- Frequent winter 'bronchitis'
- Wheeze
- Weight ↓
- Waking at night
- Ankle swelling
- Fatigue

**Signs:** Possible signs in the late stages:
- Hyperinflated chest ± poor chest expansion on inspiration
- ↓ crico-sternal distance
- Hyper-resonant chest with ↓ cardiac dullness on percussion
- Use of accessory muscles
- Paradoxical movement of lower ribs
- Tachypnoea
- Wheeze or quiet breath sounds
- Pursing of lips on expiration (pursed lip breathing)
- Peripheral oedema
- Cyanosis
- ↑ JVP
- Cachexia

**Spirometry[£]:** Predicts prognosis but not disability/quality of life – Table 5.17.

## Non-drug therapy:
- Educate the patient and family about the disease, medication and self-help strategies.
- **Smoking cessation:** Most important method to improve outcome[£].
- **Vaccination:** All patients with COPD should have influenza and pneumococcal vaccination[£].
- **Exercise:** Lack of exercise ↓ $FEV_1$. Pulmonary rehabilitation is of proven benefit – refer via respiratory physician if available locally.
- **Nutrition:** Weight ↓ in obese patients improves exercise tolerance. Consider food supplements if cachexic.

**Table 5.16 MRC Dyspnoea Scale**

| Grade | Degree of breathlessness related to physical activity |
|-------|--------------------------------------------------------|
| 1 | Not troubled by breathlessness except on strenuous exercise |
| 2 | Short of breath when hurrying or walking up a slight hill |
| 3 | Walks slower than contemporaries on level ground because of breathlessness or has to stop for breath when walking at own pace |
| 4 | Stops for breath after walking about 100m or after a few minutes on level ground |
| 5 | Too breathless to leave the house or breathless on dressing/ undressing |

Reproduced with permission of the Medical Research Council.

**Table 5.17 Severity of COPD and expected clinical picture**

| Severity | Clinical state | Spirometry |
|----------|----------------|------------|
| Mild | Cough but little or no breathlessness. No abnormal signs. No ↑ use of services | $FEV_1$ 50–80% predicted |
| Moderate | Breathlessness, wheeze on exertion, cough ± sputum and some abnormal signs. Usually known to GP – intermittent complaints | $FEV_1$ 30–49% predicted |
| Severe | SOBOE. Marked wheeze and cough. Usually other signs too. Likely to be known to GP and hospital consultant with frequent problems/admissions | $FEV_1$ <30% predicted |

**Drug therapy:** Document effects of each drug treatment on symptoms, quality of life and lung function as tried – Figure 5.7.

**Palliative measures:** If standard treatments (e.g. bronchodilators, antibiotics, corticosteroids and/or oxygen therapy) become less effective and do not relieve symptoms, consider palliative treatments.

- *Breathlessness:* Oral morphine e.g Oramorph® 2.5–5mg 4 hourly often eases resistant breathlessness – titrate dose upwards as needed. For patients with $CO_2$ retention, careful monitoring is vital, and frequency of dosing may need to be reduced. Prescribe a laxative concurrently.
- *Anxiety:* Being breathless is frightening. Anxiety can exacerbate breathlessness. A low dose benzodiazepine can be helpful e.g. lorazepam 1–2mg sl prn. Do not use diazepam as, even at low doses, it accumulates due to its long half life.

## Figure 5.7 Drug management of COPD

Diagnosis of COPD

Start short acting bronchodilator for relief of breathlessness
$\beta_2$ agonist e.g. salbutamol 100–200mcg (1–2 puffs) as needed or
anticholinergic e.g. ipratropium 20–40mcg 3–4x/d.
Both ↑FEV$_1$ and ↓ breathlessness

Poor symptom control

Combine short acting bronchodilators from different therapeutic groups
e.g. salbutamol and ipratropium

Poor symptom control

Consider a long acting bronchodilator ($\beta_2$ agonist or anticholinergic)
e.g. salmeterol 50mcg bd

Poor symptom control

Consider using a combination of a long-acting bronchodilator and inhaled
corticosteroid e.g. beclometasone 200mcg bd. Discontinue if no benefit
after 4 wk.

Poor symptom control

Consider adding SR theophylline (250–500mg bd–monitor plasma
levels and interactions)

Refer

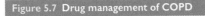
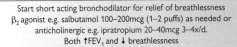
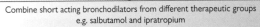
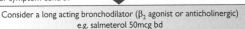

Notes:
- Phosphodiesterase type 4 inhibitors (e.g. cilomilast) – insufficient evidence of effectiveness.
- Tiotropium is a long-acting anticholinergic bronchodilator. Its place in management is not yet established.
- Antibiotics have a role in treatment of acute exacerbations of COPD. No evidence that helpful as prophylaxis.
- Oral steroids are used in the treatment of acute exacerbations. Avoid long term oral steroids if possible. Occasionally necessary for severe COPD.

| GMS Contract | | | |
|---|---|---|---|
| COPD 1 | The practice can produce a register of patients with COPD | 3 points | |
| COPD 12 | % of all patients with COPD diagnosed after 01/04/08 in whom the diagnosis had been confirmed by post bronchodilation spirometry | 5 points | 40–80% |
| COPD 10 | % of COPD patients with a record of $FEV_1$ in the previous 15mo. | 7 points | 40–70% |
| COPD 13 | % of patients with COPD who have had a review, undertaken by a healthcare professional, including an assessment of breathlessness using the MRC dyspnoea score in the preceding 15 mo. | 9 points | 50–90% |
| COPD 8 | % of COPD patients who have had influenza vaccine in the preceding 1st September – 31st March | 6 points | 40–85% |

Influenza and pneumococcal vaccination may be administered to at risk patients as a directed enhanced service (📖 p.266)

## Essential reading:

RCP/NICE. National clinical guideline on management of chronic obstructive pulmonary disease in adults in primary and secondary care (2004). *Thorax* 59 (Suppl.1): 1–232.

## Patient support:

British Lung Foundation ☎ 08458 50 20 20
🖥 www.lunguk.org

**Long-term oxygen therapy (LTOT):** *Only* prescribe after evaluation by a respiratory physician. Refer patients with:

- Severe airflow obstruction (FEV$_1$ <30% – consider if 30–49%)
- Cyanosis
- Polycythaemia
- Peripheral oedema
- ↑ JVP
- Hypoxaemia (oxygen saturation ≤92% breathing air)

Treatment for >15h./d. ↑ survival and quality of life. Ambulatory oxygen therapy can ↑ exercise tolerance in some patients. Always warn patients about the fire risks of having pure oxygen in their home.

**Acute exacerbations of COPD:** Worsening of previous stable condition. 30% have no identifiable cause – other causes include:

- *Infections:* viral upper and lower respiratory tract infections e.g. common cold, influenza; bacterial lower respiratory tract infections.
- *Pollutants* e.g. nitrous oxide, sulphur dioxide, ozone.

**Differential diagnosis:**

- Pneumonia
- LVF/pulmonary oedema
- Lung cancer
- Pleural effusion
- Recurrent aspiration
- Pneumothorax
- PE
- Upper airway obstruction

**Investigations:**

- *Pulse oximetry:* If available can be used as a measure of severity (saturation ≤92% breathing air suggests hypoxaemia – consider admission) and to monitor progress.
- *CXR:* If diagnostic doubt and/or to exclude other causes of symptoms.
- *Sputum culture:* Not recommended routinely in the community[G].

**Management:** Decide whether to admit – Table 5.18

**Home treatment of acute exacerbations:**

- *Add or ↑ bronchodilators.* Consider this option if inhaler device and technique are appropriate.
- *Start antibiotics:* Use broad spectrum antibiotic e.g. erythromycin 250–500mg qds if sputum becomes more purulent *or* clinical signs of pneumonia *or* consolidation on CXR.
- *Oral corticosteroids:* Start early in the course of the exacerbation if ↑ breathlessness which interferes with daily activities. Dosage – 30mg/d. prednisolone for 1–2wk. Consider osteoporosis prophylaxis with a bisphosphonate if frequent courses are required.

**Table 5.18** Deciding whether to treat acute exacerbations at home or in hospital. The more features in the 'treat in hospital column', the more likely the need for admission unless considered a terminal event

| Factor | Treat at home | Treat in hospital[*] |
|---|---|---|
| Ability to cope at home | Yes | No |
| Breathlessness | Mild | Severe |
| General condition | Good | Poor – deteriorating |
| Level of activity | Good | Poor/confined to bed |
| Cyanosis | No | Yes |
| Worsening peripheral oedema | No | Yes |
| Level of consciousness | Normal | Impaired |
| Already receiving LTOT | No | Yes |
| Social circumstances | Good | Living alone/not coping |
| Acute confusion | No | Yes |
| Rapid rate of onset | No | Yes |
| Significant co-morbidity (e.g. cardiac disease, IDDM) | No | Yes |
| Changes on CXR (if available) | No | Present |

*Hospital-at-home schemes and assisted discharge schemes are a suitable alternative.

Reproduced from *Thorax* (2004) **59**(Suppl 1), pp. 1–232, with permission of BMJ Publishing Group.

# Advanced heart failure

Heart failure is the common end-stage of a variety of heart diseases. Unlike cancer, pain is not usually a major problem, but oedema and breathlessness through fluid overload is often a dominant feature. In most other respects, management is similar.

## Signs:
- Cachexia and muscle wasting
- ↑ respiratory rate ± cyanosis
- ↑ pulse rate ± pulsus alternans
- Cardiomegaly and displaced apex beat ± right ventricular heave
- ↑ JVP
- 3rd heart sound
- Basal crepitations ± pleural effusions and/or wheeze
- Pitting oedema of the ankles
- Hepatomegaly ± jaundice
- Ascites

## Complications:
- Arrhythmias – especially AF and VT
- Stroke or peripheral embolus
- DVT/PE
- Malabsorption
- Hepatic congestion/dysfunction
- Muscle wasting

**Prognosis:** Progressive deterioration to death. Up to 50% die suddenly – probably due to arrhythmias. *Mortality:*
- Mild/moderate heart failure – 20–30% 1y. mortality.
- Severe heart failure – >50% 1y. mortality.

A number of factors correlate with the prognosis:
- *Clinical:* the worse the patient's symptoms the worse the prognosis.
- *Haemodynamics:* the lower the cardiac index, stroke volume and ejection fraction, the worse the prognosis.
- *Biochemical:* strong inverse correlations with certain endocrine markers; and hyponatraemia is associated with a poorer prognosis.
- *Arrhythmias:* frequent ventricular ectopics or VT on ambulatory ECG indicate a poor prognosis.

## Non-drug measures:
- *Educate* – about the disease, current/expected symptoms and need for treatment. Discuss prognosis. Support with written information.
- *Discuss ways to make life easier* e.g. benefits, mobility aids, blue disability parking badge. Consider referral to social services for assessment for home modification ± services such as home care.
- *Diet* – ensure adequate calories (consider carlorie and vitamin supplements), small frequent meals, ↓ salt, ↓ weight if obese, restrict alcohol (though a small amount is beneficial).
- *Lifestyle measures* – smoking cessation; regular exercise.
- *Restrict fluid intake* – if severe heart failure restrict intake to <1500ml/d.
- *Vaccination* – influenza and pneumococcal vaccination[f].
- *Assess for depression* – common among patients with heart failure.

## Advice for patients: Patient experiences of chronic heart failure

### Breathlessness

'When I started getting alarmingly puffy, and especially alarming was getting breathless lying down in bed and I thought well this is not right, this is something wrong ... I went down to the local doctor ... and she decided to send me for a scan in the hospital.'

'Shortness of breath, you know, wanting to do things more or less like out of the ordinary, such as gardening, you know. Out of my ordinary scope, of course, I can't, because shortness of breath steps in and you can feel your heart sometimes, you know? You can feel it's there, it starts to ... you can feel the beat. And when I start to feel the beat then I know it's time to slow down.'

'If I'm lying flat then often I'll wake up probably breathless but maybe with a coughing attack. Coughing is a real problem for me when I'm flat. And I wake up also early in the morning, when I wake up 4 o'clock, 5 o'clock, 6 o'clock but I'll often to off to sleep again for a bit, but I'm always up by 7. Just to go to bed and have an interrupted nights sleep and wake up at 8 o'clock would be delicious, but it isn't happening, and we are nearly two years in now, so I don't think it's going to come back.'

### Work tolerance:

'I can do half as much as I used to. I can't do hard work now, or heavy work, no. I can do light work, and I could go all day, but I couldn't do hard work, no.'

### Tiredness:

'It's not a "tired" tired where you want to go to bed and sleep, it's a weary tired as if everything is an effort. It's a tired where you don't want to go to bed and sleep, you just want to...I don't know...it's like a weary tired, that's the only way I can describe it really. I can't say it's a "go to sleep" tired. I don't really know, it's just an "I must sit down" tired, "I just can't take another step" tired.'

## Information for patients and their carers

**British Heart Foundation** ☎ 0300 330 3311 ▢ www.bhf.org.uk
**Healthtalkonline** Database of personal and health experiences: heart failure ▢ www.healthtalkonline.org

Patient experiences of heart failure are reproduced from the Healthtalkonline database of patient experience ▢ www. healthtalkonline.org

## Further information:

**NICE**. Chronic heart failure (2003) ▢ www.nice.org.uk
**Davis et al.** ABC of Heart Failure (2006). BMJ Books. ISBN 0727916440

## Drug treatment:

*Aims to:*
- Improve symptoms – diuretics, digoxin and ACE inhibitors[£] *and*
- Improve survival – ACE inhibitors[£], β-blockers, oral nitrates plus hydralazine, spironolactone.

**Algorithm for drug treatment of heart failure:** Figure 5.8

**Palliative measures:** Use to supplement active treatment aimed at controlling symptoms:
- Consider oxygen therapy – weigh up pros and cons – fire risk, inconvenience, upheaval of installation vs. improvement in breathing. Refer as necessary.
- Consider opioids – Oral morphine e.g Oramorph® 2.5–5mg 4 hourly often eases the sensation of resistant breathlessness – titrate dose upwards as needed. For patients with renal failure, careful monitoring is vital, and frequency of dosing may need to be reduced. Prescribe a laxative concurrently.

**Monitoring:** Review as required. Check:
- *Clinical state* – functional capacity, fluid status, cardiac rhythm, cognitive and nutritional status, mood.
- *Medication* – ensure drug record is up to date, review compliance and side effects, change drugs if clinical circumstances/best practice alter.
- *Blood* – U&E and creatinine.

| GMS Contract | | | |
|------|-----------------------------------------------------------|-----------|---------|
| HF 1 | The practice can produce a register of patients with heart failure | 4 points | |
| HF 2 | % of patients with a diagnosis of heart failure (diagnosed after 1.4.2006) which has been confirmed by an echocardiogram or by specialist assessment | 6 points | 40–90% |
| HF 3 | % of patients with a current diagnosis of heart failure due to left ventricular dysfunction who are currently treated with an ACE inhibitor or Angiotensin Receptor Blocker, who can tolerate therapy and for whom there is no contraindication | 10 points | 40–80% |

QoF points may also be available for screening for depression in patients with heart disease, secondary prevention of cardiovascular disease, and treatment of hypertension, and diabetes.

Influenza and pneumonococcal vaccination may be administered to high risk patients as a directed enhanced service (📖 p.266).

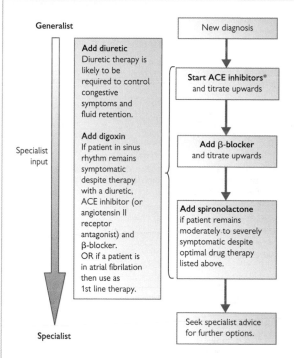

Figure 5.8 NICE algorithm for pharmacological treatment of symptomatic heart failure due to left ventricular systolic dysfunction

*If ACE inhibitor is not tolerated (e.g. due to severe cough) consider an angiotensin II receptor antagonist.

Reproduced from *Chronic Heart Failure: Management of Chronic Heart Failure in Adults in Primary and Secondary Care* (2003) with permission of NICE. Full document available at www.nice.org.uk

175

### Further information:
**NICE**. Chronic heart failure (2003) www.nice.org.uk
**SIGN**. Diagnosis and treatment of heart failure due to left ventricular systolic dysfunction (1999) www.sign.ac.uk

**Advice for patients: Information and support**

**British Heart Foundation** ☎ 0845 0708 070 www.bhf.org.uk

# Motor neurone disease (MND)

Motor neurone disease is a degenerative disorder of unknown cause affecting motor neurones in the spinal cord, brain stem and motor cortex.

Prevalence in the UK ~4.5/100,000 population ♂:♀ ≈3:2. Peak age of onset ≈60y. 10% have a FH.

**Patterns of disease:** There are three recognized patterns of MND:
- *Amyotrophic lateral sclerosis (ALS)* (50%) – combined LMN wasting and UMN hyperreflexia.
- *Progressive muscular atrophy* (25%) – anterior horn cell lesions affecting distal before proximal muscles. Better prognosis than ALS.
- *Progressive bulbar palsy* (25%) – loss of function of brainstem motor nuclei (LMN lesions) resulting in weakness of the tongue, muscles of chewing/swallowing and facial muscles.

**Clinical picture:** Combination of progressive upper and/or lower motor neurone signs affecting >1 limb or a limb and the bulbar muscles.

## Symptoms/signs:
- Stumbling (spastic gait, foot-drop)
- Tiredness
- Muscle wasting
- Weak grip
- Weakness of skeletal muscles
- Cramp
- Fasciculation of skeletal muscles
- Fasciculation of the tongue
- Difficulty with speech (particularly slurring, hoarseness or nasal or quiet speech)
- Difficulty with swallowing
- Aspiration pneumonia.

⚠ MND *never* affects external ocular movements (cranial nerves III, IV and VI). There is *never* any sensory loss.

**Management:** Refer to neurology for exclusion of other causes of the symptoms and confirmation of diagnosis. MND is incurable and progressive. Death usually results from ventilatory failure 3–5y. after diagnosis.

## Drug therapy:
- Riluzole (50mg bd) is the only drug treatment licensed in the UK.
- Evidence suggests that it may extend time to mechanical ventilation for patients with ALS. It may also slow functional decline[N], but effects on survival are unproven.
- It should be initiated by a specialist with experience of MND[N].
- Monitoring of liver function is essential – monthly for the first 3mo.; then 3 monthly for 9mo.; then annually thereafter.

### Support:
- Involve relevant agencies early e.g. DN, social services, carer groups, self-help groups.
- Apply for all relevant benefits (📖 p.238–249).
- Discuss the future, and the patient's wishes for the time when they become incapacitated, with patient and carer(s).
- Regular review to help overcome any new problems encountered is helpful for patients and carers.

### Symptom relief:
- *Spasticity:* baclofen, tizanidine and botulinum toxin may all be effective.
- *Drooling:* Try propantheline 15–30mg tds po or amitriptyline 25–50mg tds po or atropine eye drops 9 drops po.
- *Dysphagia:* Blend food, discuss nasogastric tubes/PEG (📖 p.112).
- *Depression:* Common – reassess support, consider drug treatment and/or counselling.
- *Joint pains:* Provide analgesia.
- *Respiratory failure:* Prophylactic antibiotics may prevent infection – appropriateness depends on clinical state. Discuss tracheostomy/ventilation – weigh pros and cons of prolongation of life vs. prolongation of discomfort. In some cases for example for patients suffering nightmares or morning headache – limited ventilation (e.g. non-invasive positive pressure ventilation at night) may be appropriate even if ventilation is not wanted to prolong life.

**Vaccination[£]:** Offer influenza and pneumococcal vaccination to all MND patients.

### Further information:
**NICE:** Riluzole for motor neurone disease – full guidance (2001 and review 2004). 🖳 www.nice.org.uk

---

#### Advice for patients: Support for patients and carers

**Motor Neurone Disease Association** ☎ Helpline: 08457 626262
🖳 www.mndassociation.org
**Brain and Spine Foundation** ☎ 0808 808 1000
🖳 www.brainandspine.org.uk

---

#### GMS Contract

Influenza and pneumococcal vaccination may be offered by GMS practices as a directed enhanced service – 📖 p.266.

# Multiple sclerosis (MS)

Multiple sclerosis (MS) is a chronic disabling neurological disease due to an autoimmune process of unknown cause. Characterized by formation of patches of demyelination ("plaques") throughout the brain and spinal cord. There is no peripheral nerve involvement.

It is the most common neurological disorder of young adults with a lifetime risk of 1:1000. Peak age of onset is 20-40y. ♀:♂ ≈ 2:1. There is a marked geographical variation – prevalence ↑ with latitude.

**Presentation:** Depends on the area of CNS affected. Take a careful history – although a patient usually presents with a single symptom, history may reveal other episodes that have gone unheralded. Isolated neurological deficits are never diagnostic. The hallmark of MS is a series of neurological deficits distributed in time and space not attributable to other causes. Predominant areas of demyelination are optic nerve, cervical cord and periventricular areas.

## Common features:

- Pain on eye movement (optic neuritis)
- Visual disturbance – ↓, blurring or double vision
- ↓ balance
- ↓ coordination
- Sensory disturbance (e.g. numbness, tingling)
- Pain (e.g. trigeminal neuralgia)
- Fatigue
- Depression
- Transverse myelitis
- Problems with speech (e.g. slurred or slow)
- Bladder problems (e.g. frequency, urgency, incontinence)
- Constipation
- Sexual dysfunction (e.g. impotence)
- Cognitive changes (e.g. loss of concentration, memory problems)
- Dysphagia

🛈 Symptoms may be worsened by heat or exercise.

## Prognosis:

- **Benign MS** (rare): Few mild attacks and then complete recovery. There is no deterioration over time and no permanent disability.
- **Relapsing-remitting MS (RRMS):** 90% patients. Episodes of sudden ↑ in neurological symptoms or development of new neurological symptoms with virtually complete recovery after 4-6 wk.. With time remissions become less complete and residual disability accumulates.
- **Secondary progressive MS (SPMS):** After ~ 10y. about ½ the patients with relapsing-remitting disease begin a continuous downward progression which may also include acute relapses.
- **Primary progressive MS (PPMS):** 10% patients. Steady progression from the outset with increasing disability.

**Management:** If suspected, refer to neurology for confirmation of diagnosis and support from specialist neurological rehabilitation.

**Disease modifying drugs:** ↓ frequency and/or severity of relapses by ~ 30% and slow course of the disease. Options are β-interferon (for RRMS and SPMS) and glatiramer (for RRMS only). Prescription must be consultant led under the NHS risk sharing scheme – Table 16.11.

### Table 5.19 Indications for β-interferon and glatiramer[N]

|  | β-interferon | Glatiramer |
|---|---|---|
| Age | ≥ 18y. | ≥ 18y. |
| Contraindications | No contraindications | No contraindications |
| Walking distance | RRMS: Can walk ≥ 100m without assistance<br>SPMS: Can walk ≥ 10m without assistance | RRMS: Can walk ≥ 100m without assistance |
| Relapses | RRMS: ≥ 2 clinically significant relapses in the last year<br>SPMS: Minimal ↑ in disability due to gradual progression and ≥ 2 disabling relapses in the past 2y. | RRMS: ≥ 2 clinically significant relapses in the last year |
| Stop if: | • Intolerable side effects<br>• Pregnant or planning pregnancy<br>• ≥2 disabling relapses within a year<br>• Inability to walk (± help) persisting ≥ 6 mo.<br>• 2° progression with observable ↑ in disability over 6 mo. | • Intolerable side effects<br>• Pregnant or planning pregnancy<br>• ≥2 disabling relapse within a year<br>• Inability to walk (± help) persisting ≥ 6 mo.<br>• 2° progression |

**179**

**Natalizumab:** monoclonal antibody for treatment of highly active relapsing-remitting MS, despite treatment with β-interferon, or rapidly evolving severe relapsing-remitting MS. Prescription must be consultant led. Associated with an ↑ risk of opportunistic infection and progressive multifocal leucoencephalopathy (PML). If new/worsening neurological symptoms/signs refer to neurology immediately to exclude PML

### GMS Contract

Influenza and pneumococcal vaccination may be offered by GMS practices as a directed enhanced service – 📖 p.266

Specialized services for patients with MS can be provided as a national enhanced service – 📖 p.268

**Acute relapses:** Treat episodes causing distressing symptoms or ↑ limitation with high-dose steroids e.g. prednisolone 500mg–2g od po for 3–5d. Alternatively, refer for high-dose IV steroids. Refer to specialist neurological rehabilitation if there is a residual deficit. If frequent courses of steroids consider osteoporosis prophylaxis.

**Symptom relief:** Specialist multidisciplinary support is essential.

**Motor impairment:** Aim to maintain physical independence:
- Involve physiotherapy – often only 2–3 visits are needed.
- Involve OT – a task-oriented approach is used (e.g. learning how to dress). Can also supply/advise on aids and appliances e.g. velcro fasteners, wheelchairs, adapted cutlery etc.
- Refer for social services OT assessment if aids, equipment or adaptations are needed for the home.
- Refer for home care services as necessary.
- Give information about driving (📖 p.226) and employment (📖 p.222).

**Spasticity ± muscle and joint contractures:** Treat with physiotherapy (usually involving exercise ± splinting) ± drugs. Anti-spasticity drugs include dantrolene (25mg od), baclofen (5mg tds or rarely through a pump) and tizanidine (2mg od). Botulinum toxin can be directed at specific muscles. Refer via the specialist rehabilitation team.

**Communication problems:** Speech therapy assessment is vital. Consider support via dysphasia groups and communication aids e.g. simple pointing board (take advice from speech therapy and OT).

**Poor vision:** Refer to an optician in the first instance. If corrected vision is still poor refer for ophthalmology review.

**Respiratory infections:** Common. Treat with antibiotics unless in terminal stages of disease. Advise pneumococcal and influenza vaccination[£].

**Venous thromboembolism:** Common but clinically apparent in <5%. Ensure adequate hydration and encourage mobility. Consider use of aspirin 75–150mg od and compression stockings if immobile. Prophylactic anticoagulation does not improve outcome.

**Skin breakdown:** *Prevented by:* positioning; mobilization; good skin care; management of incontinence; pressure relieving aids (e.g. special mattresses/cushions). Involve community nursing services.

**Bladder problems**
- *UTI:* If suspected check urine dipstick ± send MSU for M, C&S and start antibiotics. If >3 proven UTIs in 1y. refer to specialist incontinence service or urology for further assessment.
- *Incontinence:* 📖 p.128.
- *Nocturia:* desmopressin 100–400mcgm po or 10–40mcgm intranasally nocte may be helpful.
- *Urgency:* Modify environment e.g. provide commode; try anticholinergic e.g. tolterodine 2mg bd or oxybutynin 5mg tds. If not settling refer for specialist assessment.

Consider:
- Is it due to an unrelated disease? e.g. change in bowel habit might indicate bowel cancer.
- Is it due to an incidental infection? e.g. UTI, chest infection.
- Is it due to a relapse? e.g. acute relapse in MS.
- Is it due to a side effect of treatment? e.g. acute confusion due to steroids or drowsiness due to opioids.
- Is it part of a gradual progression?

Treat any cause of deterioration identified. If no cause is found, consider re-referring for specialist review and/or referring to the multidisciplinary rehabilitation team involved with the patient.

**Advice for patients: Sexual and personal relationships**

Problems are common. Useful information sheets and a helpline are available at ☎ 0707 499 3527 🖥 www.outsiders.org.uk

*Bowel problems*
- *Dysphagia:* Common. Fluids are more difficult to swallow than semisolids. Formal assessment by trained staff is essential. Feeding through a N-G tube or PEG may be needed long or short term. In terminal disease weigh provision of nutrition against prolongation of poor-quality life.
- *Constipation:* Difficulty with defaecation or bowels open <2x/wk. – ↑ fluid intake and ↑ fibre in diet. If no improvement use po laxative ± regular suppositories/enemas.
- *Incontinence:* Exclude overflow due to constipation.

*Fatigue:* Consider and treat factors that might be responsible:
- Depression
- Chronic pain
- Disturbed sleep
- Poor nutrition

*Action:* Review support, diet and medication, encourage graded aerobic exercise, consider a trial of amantadine 200mg/d. to improve symptoms[N].

**Depression and anxiety:** Common. Non-specific symptoms may be the first presentation of depression or an anxiety disorder. Fatigue, sleep disturbance, and unexplained pain are frequent presentations of underlying depression. Many symptoms of MS are similar to symptoms of depression – if suspected, a trial of antidepressants is worthwhile.

**Emotionalism:** If the patient cries (or laughs) with minimal provocation, consider emotionalism – impairment in the control of crying. Reassure.

**Pain:** 60% of patients with MS have chronic pain – 40% of those say their pain is not controlled. Most pain arises from, ↓ mobility. *Other causes include:* pre-morbid disease (e.g. osteoarthritis), central pain due to neurological damage and neuropathic pain.
- Neuropathic and central pain – treat with tricyclic antidepressants or anticonvulsants – 📖 p.40.
- Musculoskeletal pain – Try NSAIDs ± paracetamol ± a weak opioid ± physiotherapy. Splints, massage and TENS/acupuncture may also be helpful.

❶ Trials of cannabis/cannabinoids in treatment of MS pain are in advanced stages – meanwhile many patients use illicit supplies to help ease their pain.

**Diet:** Supplementing the diet with 17–23gd. of linoleic *acid* (a polyunsaturated fat) may ↓ progression of disability[N]. Rich sources of linoleic acid include sunflower, corn, soya and safflower oils.

## Support:
- Involve relevant agencies early e.g. DN, social services, carer groups, self-help groups.
- Apply for all relevant benefits (📖 p.238–249).
- Discuss the future, and the patient's wishes for the time when they become incapacitated, with patient and carer(s).
- Regular review to help overcome any new problems encountered is helpful for patients and carers.

**Carers:** 📖 p.250

**Benefits:** 📖 p.238–249

**Driving:** 📖 p.226

### Further information:

**NICE/RCP.** Diagnosis and management of multiple sclerosis in primary and secondary care (2003) 🖳 www.nice.org.uk

**DoH** HSC 2002/004 Cost-effective provision of disease-modifying therapies for people with MS 🖳 www.dh.gov.uk

**MS Society** A guide to MS for GPs and primary care teams (2006) 🖳 www.mssociety.org.uk

# Human immunodeficiency virus (HIV)

Advanced HIV infection is accompanied by immunosuppression or acquired immune deficiency syndrome (AIDS – if CD4 count <200cells/mm$^3$). Patients are at risk from:

- Opportunistic infections (e.g. pneumococcal infection, TB, CMV, HSV, *Pneumocystis carinii*, toxoplasmosis and cryptosporidial diarrhoea) *and*
- AIDS-associated malignancies (e.g. Kaposi's sarcoma – usually of lung or skin, lymphoma).

**Death from HIV:** Is due to multiple causes, including chronic incurable systemic infections, malignancies, neurological disease, wasting and malnutrition, and multisystem failure.

**Management of HIV infection$^G$:** Specialist treatment is essential.

**Antiviral drugs:** 3 groups:
- Nucleoside analogues (e.g. Zidovudine).
- Non-nucleoside reverse transcriptase inhibitors (e.g. Nevirapine).
- Protease inhibitors (e.g. Indinavir).

Highly active antiretroviral therapy (HAART) is a combination of ≥3 drugs with ≥1 drug penetrating the blood–brain barrier. Many of the drugs have severe side effects. Adherence to therapy is essential to avoid resistance. Patients who present with clinical manifestations of HIV, CD4 counts <350cells/mm$^3$ or viral loads >30,000 copies are considered for HAART. Treatment failure requires switching or increasing therapy with at least 2 new drugs.

**Prophylaxis against opportunistic infection:** Patients with low CD4 counts are started on prophylactic antibiotics:
- <200cells/mm$^3$ – *Pneumocystis carinii* (co-trimoxazole).
- <100cells/mm$^3$ – toxoplasmosis (co-trimoxazole).
- <50cells/mm$^3$ – *Mycobacterium avium* (azithromycin).

**Psychological support and palliative care:**
- Perhaps the most important role of the GP and community services.
- Patients often lack the support offered for most other terminal illnesses as HIV infection remains stigmatized, usually involves young patients and often affects people in marginalized/minority groups.
- HIV differs from most other terminal illnesses as other family members/partners are often infected too. Patients may have seen their peers die from HIV infection.

**Management of specific problems:** Table 5.20

**Other common problems:** Treat symptomatically.
- Wasting, weakness, and dependency
- Slowing of mental functions including AIDS-related dementia
- Loss of libido
- Premature greying and loss of hair
- Molluscum contagiosum
- Progressive visual loss from retinitis
- Incontinence (especially faecal – may be 2° to diarrhoea)

## Table 5.20 Specific symptoms in palliative care of HIV patients and management solutions

| Problem | Management |
|---------|-----------|
| Pain | Treat with analgesia 📖 p.14 |
| | Exclude underlying causes: |
| | *Oropharyngeal* – *Candida*, herpes viruses (HSV, CMV, VZ), apthous-type ulcers, malignancy, gingivitis, tooth abscesses |
| | *Retrosternal* – Oesophageal *Candida*, infection with CMV or HSV, giant oesophageal ulcers, reflux oesophagitis, Pneumocystis carinii pneumonia |
| | *Headache* – Toxoplasmosis, cryptococcal meningitis, cerebral lymphoma |
| | *Abdominal* – Diarrhoea ± infection, AIDS-related sclerosing cholangitis, malignancy (e.g. Kaposi's sarcoma, lymphoma), drugs (e.g. clarithromycin), constipation |
| | *Perianal and perineal* – HSV (very common, needs high index of suspicion), *Candida*, excoriation of skin due to diarrhoea |
| Cough | Send sputum for M, C&S and virology/mycology |
| | Consider CXR to exclude Karopsi's sarcoma, TB and other chest infections |
| | Treat specific conditions when appropriate. Consider decongestants |
| Anorexia, nausea, and vomiting | Dietary advice – small meals frequently |
| | Exclude constipation |
| | Review medication |
| | Review *Candida* treatment |
| | Consider antiemetics – 📖 p.114 |
| Diarrhoea | Check stool sample for M, C&S to exclude treatable infective causes: *Salmonella*, *Giardia*, *Campylobacter*, *Clostridium difficile*, CMV |
| | Exclude constipation and drug causes |
| | Consider malabsorption as a cause – pancreatin supplements may help |
| | Diarrhoea caused by untreatable infection e.g. due to *Crypto-sporidium* or *Microsporidium* or diarrhoea for which no cause can be found can be difficult to control – consider opioids and/or octreotide |
| Malaise, weakness, pyrexia | Consider drug effects. A trial of steroids may be worthwhile |
| Dermatitis/ pruritus | Treat the cause where possible e.g. |
| | ● Iron supplements for iron-deficiency anaemia |
| | ● Anti-scabies treatment |
| | ● Topical or systemic antibiotics for folliculitis |
| | Otherwise treat with emollients and antipruritics (e.g. chlorphenamine 4mg qds prn). Consider a trial of topical steroid cream bd |

185

---

### Advice for patients: Information and support

NAM Aidsmap 🖥 www.aidsmap.com
National AIDS Helpline ☎ 0800 567 123 (24h. helpline)
Terrence Higgins Trust ☎ 0845 1221 200 🖥 www.tht.org.uk

**Control of infection:** There is an extremely low risk of infection to household contacts and healthcare workers. HIV is present in blood and bodily fluids – advise carers to wear gloves when there is a risk of direct contact with these fluids. Gloves are not needed for normal examination or casual household contact. Linen and cutlery should be washed as normal. Spillages should be cleaned up with household bleach.

**Needle-stick injury:** Exposure is significant if the source is HIV +ve, the material is blood or another infectious body fluid (semen, amniotic fluid, genital secretions, CSF) and exposure is caused by inoculation (risk transmission 1:300 if HIV +ve source) or by a splash onto a mucous membrane (risk transmission 1:3000).

⚠ *Immediate action:* Irrigate site of exposure with running water; establish potential risk of HIV – history of HIV infection and (if possible) blood sample from the source and victim. Refer to A&E immediately for instigation of HIV prevention policy.

## Further information:

**British HIV Association**. HIV treatment guidelines (2006) ⊡ www.bhiva.org
**Health Protection Agency (HPA)**. HIV ⊡ www.hpa.org.uk
**DoH**. Winning ways: reducing healthcare associated infection in England (2004) ⊡ www.dh.gov.uk
Medical Foundation for AIDS and Sexual Health HIV in primary care (2004 and revision 2005) ⊡ www.medfash.org.uk

# The last 48 hours

It is notoriously difficult to predict when death will occur. Avoid the trap of predicting or making a guess unless absolutely pushed to do so. Talk in terms of 'days' or 'weeks'. For example:

'When we see someone deteriorating from week to week we are often talking in terms of weeks; when that deterioration is from day to day then we are usually talking in terms of days, but everyone is different.'

## Symptoms and signs of death approaching:

- Day-by-day deterioration
- Gaunt appearance
- Profound weakness – needs assistance with all care, may be bedbound
- Difficulty swallowing medicines
- ↓ intake of food and fluids
- Drowsy or ↓ cognition – often unable to co-operate with carers

## Goals of treatment in the last 48h.:

- Try to ensure patients are comfortable – physically, emotionally, and spiritually.
- Make the end of life peaceful and dignified – what is dignified for one patient may not be for another – ask.
- Support patients and carers so that the experience of death for those left behind is as positive as it can be.

**Patients' wishes:** Dying is a unique event for each individual. Helping to explore a patient's wishes about death and dying should not be a discussion left to the last 24h.

## Advance directives/living wills: 📖 p.225

**Different cultures:** Different religious and cultural groups have different approaches to the dying process. It is important to be sensitive to cultural and religious beliefs. If in doubt, ask a family member. You are more likely to cause offence by not asking than by asking.

**Assessment of a patient's needs:** Try to discover which problems are causing the patient/carers most concern and address those concerns where possible. Patients often under-report their symptoms and families/carers may misinterpret symptoms.

**Physical examination:** Keep examination to a minimum to avoid unnecessary interference. Check:
- Sites of discomfort/pain suggested by history or non-verbal cues
- Mouth
- Bladder and bowel

**Psychological assessment:** Find out what the patient wants to know. Gently assessing how the patient feels about their disease and situation can shed light on their needs and distress.

**Investigations:** Any investigation at the end of life should have a clear and justifiable purpose (e.g. excluding a reversible condition where treatment would make the patient more comfortable). The need for investigations in the terminal stage of illness is minimal.

Death is a taboo subject and few people feel comfortable discussing it – even though it is natural, certain, and happening all around us all the time.

Opening up discussion can be liberating to patients who then may feel they are being given permission to talk about dying. Families do not like discussions about dying for fear that patients will 'give up'.

Sometimes the direct question 'Are you worried about dying?' is the most appropriate. Often patients' biggest fears are groundless and reassurance can be given. Where reassurance cannot be given it is helpful to break the fear down into constituent parts and try to sort out those aspects you can deal with.

## Common fears:
- *Fears associated with symptoms* e.g. pain will escalate to agony; breathing will stop if the patient falls asleep.
- *Emotional fears* e.g. increasing dependence on family. 'It would be better if I was out of the way.'
- *Past experience* e.g. past contact with patients who died with unpleasant symptoms.
- *Preferences about treatment or withholding treatment* e.g. 'What if nobody listens to me or they don't take my wishes seriously?'
- *Fears about morphine*
- *Death and dying* – fears of being dead and the process of dying need to be differentiated.

## Referral to specialist palliative care services:
Ideally involve specialist palliative care services before the terminal phase is reached. Referral in the terminal phase is appropriate when:
- One or more distressing symptoms prove difficult to control
- There is severe emotional distress
- There are dependent children and/or elderly vulnerable relatives involved

### Review of medication
- Comfort is the priority. Stop unnecessary medication.
- Continue analgesia, antiemetics, anxiolytics/antipsychotics and anticonvulsants.
- Diabetes can be managed with once daily insulin glargine, as needed.
- Consider alternative routes of drug administration (e.g. syringe driver, patches).
- Explain changes to relatives/carers.

**Symptom control:** Dying patients tolerate symptoms very poorly because of their weakness. Nursing care is the mainstay of treatment. GPs do have a role though:
- Ensure new problems do not develop e.g. ensure use of appropriate mattresses and measures to prevent bed sores.
- Treat specific symptoms e.g. dry mouth.
- Think ahead – discuss treatment options which might be available later e.g. use of a syringe driver, buccal, pr or transcutaneous preparations to deliver medication when/if the oral route is no longer possible, use of strong analgesia that may also have a sedative effect.
- Ensure there is a clear management plan agreed between the medical and nursing team and the patient/family members. Anticipate probable needs of the patient so that immediate response can be made when the time comes – define clearly what should be done in the event of a symptom arising/worsening; ensure drugs or equipment that may be needed are in the home.

### Terminal anguish and spiritual distress
- Characterized by overwhelming distress.
- Often related to unresolved conflict, guilt, fears, or loss of control.

### Anxiety can be increased if:
- Patients are unaware of the diagnosis, but feel that people are lying to them.
- They have certain symptoms such as breathlessness, haemorrhage and constant nausea or diarrhoea.
- Weak religious conviction – convinced believers and convinced non-believers have less anxiety.
- There are young dependant children or other dependant relatives.
- Patients have unfinished business to attend to, such as legal affairs.

**Action:** Empathic listening can itself be therapeutic. Talk to the patient, if possible, about dying and try to break down fears into component parts. Address those fears that can be dealt with. As a last resort, and after discussion with the patient (where possible) and/or relatives, consider sedation (see terminal restlessness/agitation – 📖 p.192).

*Pain* 📖 pp.12–45 and 100

*Nausea and vomiting* 📖 p.114

*Artificial hydration of the dying patient* 📖 p.89

## Advice for patients: Patient experiences

### Not wanting to be a burden:

'I don't want to be a burden to my family, that is something that's definitely out of order as far as I'm concerned. I've seen other families that have endeavoured to cope with situations of that type when they couldn't and it practically destroyed the family.'

### Choosing a place to die:

'I go back to my wife who died from cancer. One of the things she said to me was, "I know I'm dying but I want to die in my own home." And my response was, "If we can manage to bring that wish to fulfilment we will do that". And with the help of my two daughters and the local community nurses and the doctor, we managed to achieve that. It was hard work. It was very emotional but we managed to carry out her last wish.'

'I think if the cancer got bad I would like to go to a hospice. My husband is not terribly practical when it comes to looking after someone who is very ill and I think that I would like, if it came to it, I think I'd like to be in a hospice where they control the pain for you, look after you.'

### Worries about death and dying:

'Again I don't know from the doctors what is likely to happen apart from they say I will just get weaker and weaker and as more pain occurs in the bones then I will be given more painkiller.'

'My biggest problem with thinking about death is not the actual dying because I can envisage that as going to sleep and not knowing anything about it like you go in for surgery. You have the anaesthetic and you're gone and you know nothing about it and you just don't wake up. I think of death like that.'

'What worries me is what's going to happen before [death], particularly with cancer because you hear so much about the pain. I've experienced pain, I've had the pain in this breast so I have experienced pain and that side of it does worry me in wondering how I would cope with it.'

### Acceptance of dying:

'Everybody is so different. Some people can shout, some people can scream, some people are quiet, it's very different, difficult. But acceptance is a great thing. It heals the mind. You know, you didn't bring it on yourself. You didn't make yourself sick. It comes on. You don't know why. So, that's all I can say because that's all I can get from it. I accept it.'

'Life is a mixture of all sorts of things. There are sad moments and there are moments when things have gone wrong and there are things when you can be upset and angry about things, but find the positives. And rejoice in those positives and rejoice in the life that you've had. Celebrate the life that you've had and come to terms with the fact that it will ultimately end. The only difference is that you now know and some people . . . well it comes to an end and they don't know about it.'

Patient experiences are reproduced with permission from the Healthtalkonline patient experience database ▣ www.healthtalkonline.org

**Terminal restlessness:** *Causes:*

- *Pain/discomfort* – urinary retention, constipation, pain which the patient cannot tell you about, excess secretions in throat.
- *Opiate toxicity* – causes myoclonic jerking. The dose of morphine may need to be ↓ if a patient becomes uraemic.
- *Biochemical causes* – ↑ $Ca^{2+}$, uraemia – ⚠ if it has been decided not to treat abnormalities DO NOT check for them.
- *Psychological/spiritual distress.*

**Management:**

- Treat reversible causes e.g. catheterization for retention, hyoscine to dry up secretions.
- If still restless, treat with an anxiolytic to reduce the suffering both of the patient and any relatives in attendance.

*Suitable drugs:* haloperidol 1–3mg tds po; chlorpromazine 25–50mg tds po; diazepam 2–10mg tds po, midazolam (10–100mg/24h. via syringe driver or 5mg stat) or levomepromazine (50–150mg/24h. via syringe driver or 6.25mg stat).

**Excessive respiratory secretion (death rattle):** Noisy, moist breathing. Rarely distresses patients but can be very distressing for relatives in attendance.

**Management:**

- Reassure relatives that the patient is not suffering or choking.
- Try repositioning and/or tipping the bed head down (if possible) to reduce the noise.
- Treat prophylactically – it is easier to prevent secretions forming than remove accumulated secretions.

*Suitable drugs:*

- Glycopyrronium – non-sedative – give 200mcgm s/cut stat and review after 1h. If effective, give 200mcgm every 4h. by s/cut injection or 0.6–1.2mg/24h. via syringe driver.
- Hyoscine hydrobromide – sedative in high doses – give 400mcgm s/cut stat and review response after 30min. If effective, give 400–600mcgm 4–8-hourly or 0.6–2.4mg/24h. via syringe driver. If the patient is conscious and respiratory secretions are not too distressing, it may be more appropriate to use a transdermal patch, (Scopoderm® 1.5mg over 3d.) or sublingual tablets (Kwells). Dry mouth is a side effect.

**Terminal breathlessness:** Distressing symptom for patients/carers.

**Management:** Support carers in attendance and explain management.

- Diamorphine or morphine: dose depends on whether the patient is being converted from oral morphine (or an alternative opioid), to diamorphine. If no previous opioid, start diamorphine 5mg/24h. s/cut. If previously on oral morphine, divide the total 24h. dose by 3 to obtain the 24h. s/cut dose of diamorphine. ↑ dose slowly as needed.
- Midazolam 5–10mg/24h. s/cut.
- If sticky secretions, try nebulized saline ± physiotherapy.

**Drugs and dosages for use in syringe drivers:** Table 5.21, 📖 pp.194–7

Table 5.21 Drugs and dosages for use in syringe drivers for palliative care
⚠ Drugs should be mixed with water unless indicated otherwise. Seek advice from palliative care drugs in a syringe driver

| Drug (ampoule size) | Indications | Compatibility | Contraindications | Side effects | prm dose | 24h. infusion dose |
|---|---|---|---|---|---|---|
| Cyclizine (50mg/ml) | • Nausea and vomiting<br>• Mechanical bowel obstruction<br>• ↑ ICP | Can precipitate with:<br>• Dexamethasone<br>• Diamorphine (in higher doses)<br>• Metoclopramide<br>• Midazolam<br>• 0.9% sodium chloride | None in patients with advanced cancer.<br>Do not give in combination with:<br>• Metoclopramide,<br>• Levomepromazine<br>• Buscopan | • Drowsiness<br>• Dry mouth<br>• Blurred vision<br>• Hypotension<br>Injection can be painful – if injection site is inflamed, try to dilute further. | 50mg s/cut prm | 50–150mg |
| Dexa-methasone (4mg/ml) | • Nausea and vomiting<br>• Pain relief<br>• ↑ ICP<br>• Spinal cord compression<br>• Intestinal obstruction<br>• Syringe driver site reaction | Mixes with metoclopramide. Advisable to put in separate syringe but can mix with diamorphine.<br>Precipitates with:<br>• Cyclizine<br>• Midazolam<br>• Haloperidol | Diabetes – needs strict supervision of blood glucose level | • GI side effects<br>• Impaired healing<br>• ↑ appetite and weight gain<br>• Hirsutism | Not usually needed | 4–16mg<br>1mg for syringe driver site reaction |
| Diamorphine (5mg, 10mg, 30mg, 100mg, 500mg) | • Pain<br>• Dyspnoea<br>• Cough<br>• Diarrhoea | With most drugs | None – ↓ dose in renal failure | 🕮 p.34 | One sixth of total 24h. dose<br>Acts in 10–30 min. | Variable – 🕮 p.38 |

| | | | | |
|---|---|---|---|---|
| Diclofenac (75mg/3ml) | Pain (particularly musculoskeletal pain) | Incompatible with most drugs. Use in a separate syringe driver with 0.9% saline for dilution. | • Active peptic ulceration • Angioedema Caution in patients with asthma, rhinitis or urticaria. | Skin ulceration (especially with prolonged use) | 75mg s/cut bd (Do not give as well as infusion) Acts in 20–30min. | 75–150mg |
| Glycopyrronium bromide (0.2mg/ml; 0.6mg/3ml) | • Death rattle • Colic in inoperable bowel obstruction • Reduction of secretions | With most drugs | | • Tachycardia • Dry mouth | 0.2mg s/cut every 6–8h. Acts in 20–40min. | 0.6–1.2mg |
| Haloperidol (5mg/ml) | • Nausea and vomiting • Hiccup • Acute confusion/ psychotic symptoms | With most drugs | Parkinson's disease Possible CNS depression with alcohol/anxiolytics. | • Extrapyramidal symptoms • Dry mouth • Drowsiness • Difficulty in micturition • Hypotension • Blurred vision | 1.5mg od s/cut for nausea. 1.5–3mg s/cut tds for agitation (may need 5mg stat if very agitated) Acts in 10–15min. | 3–5mg Avoid doses >10mg |
| Hyoscine butylbromide (20mg/ml) | • Obstruction with colic • Death rattle • Excess secretions | With most drugs except cyclizine | • Narrow angle glaucoma • Myasthenia gravis | | 20mg s/cut every 4h. Acts in 3–5min. | 40–100mg |

Table 5.21 (Contd.)

| Drug (ampoule size) | Indications | Compatibility | Contraindications | Side effects | prn dose | 24h. infusion dose |
|---|---|---|---|---|---|---|
| Hyoscine hydrobromide (0.4mg/ml; 0.8mg/ml) | • Death rattle<br>• Colic<br>• ↓ salivation | | | • Sedation | 0.4mg every 6–8h. | 1.2–2.4mg |
| Levomepromazine (25mg/ml) | • Nausea and vomiting<br>• Insomnia<br>• Terminal agitation<br>• Intractable pain | Precipitates with dexamethasone<br>Do not use with cyclizine | • Parkinson's disease<br>• Postural hypotension<br>• Antihypertensive therapy<br>• Epilepsy<br>• Hypothyroidism<br>• Myasthenia gravis | • Sedation<br>• Postural hypotension | 6.25–12.5mg s/cut od or bd for nausea<br>Acts in 30min. | 6.25–25mg for nausea/vomiting<br>25–150mg for terminal agitation |
| Metoclopramide (10mg/2ml) | Nausea and vomiting | With most drugs | Do not give in bowel obstruction if colic.<br>Do not give with antimuscarinic drugs (e.g. cyclizine) | • Dizziness<br>• Diarrhoea<br>• Depression<br>• Extrapyramidal side effects | 10–20mg s/cut every 6h. | 60–120mg |
| Midazolam (10mg/2ml) | • Terminal agitation<br>• Epilepsy/myoclonus<br>• Hiccup<br>• Muscle spasm | With most drugs | • Drowsiness<br>• Hypotension | • Dizziness<br>• Drowsiness | 2.5–10mg s/cut every 4h.<br>Acts in 5–10min. | 10–60mg |

| Drug | Indications | Incompatibilities | Cautions/Contraindications | Side effects | prn dose | Dose |
|---|---|---|---|---|---|---|
| Octreotide<br>Specialist use only | • Intestinal obstruction and vomiting<br>• Diarrhoea<br>• Bowel fistulae | Precipitates with dexamethasone | Caution in diabetics – may cause hypoglycaemia | • Dry mouth<br>• Nausea or vomiting<br>• Anorexia<br>• Abdominal pain<br>• Flatulence | Not usually given as prn dose | 1200mcgm |
| Oxycodone (10mg/1ml; 20mg/2ml) | Pain | Incompatible with cyclizine when concentration of cyclizine is >3mg/ml (i.e. 60mg in a standard 20ml syringe). | Hypersensitivity to opioids. Severe renal impairment (creatinine clearance <10ml/min.). Concurrent administration of MAOIs or <2wk. after discontinuation. | 🕮 p.34 | One sixth of total 24h. dose<br>Acts in 10–30min. | Variable –<br>🕮 pp.29–30 |

# Chapter 6

# Complementary medicine

# Complementary medicine

In the UK ~90% of the population have tried complementary or alternative medicine (CAM) at some time. Patients commonly turn to CAM when conventional treatments can not offer a 'cure' e.g. when they have chronic pain or in palliative care situations. But, although CAM undoubtedly helps many individuals, its use remains controversial.

## Reasons for caution:

- *Lack of evidence of effectiveness:* There are many anecdotal reports and small-scale observational studies of the positive effects of complementary therapies but large scale, high quality studies tend to be −ve.
- *Lack of regulation of practitioners:* Anyone can call themselves a therapist and practice. It is always important to find a reputable practitioner with accredited training who is a member of a recognized professional body. It is also important to ensure any practitioner used carries professional indemnity insurance.
- *Lack of regulation of products:* Most complementary 'medicines' are sold as foods rather than medicines and do not hold a product licence. No licensing authority has assessed efficacy, safety or quality, and interactions with conventional medicines are unknown. Complementary medicines can, and do, cause adverse effects − just because they are natural does not mean they are safe.

## Legal position of GPs:

**Practising complementary medicine:** Conventionally trained doctors can administer any unconventional medical treatments they choose. The 'Bolam test' applies − in other words, if a doctor has undergone additional training in a complementary discipline and practises in a way that is reasonable and would be considered acceptable by a number of other medically qualified complementary practitioners, his or her actions are defensible.

## Referring patients to complementary medicine practitioners:

- *Delegation to non-medically qualified practitioner:* Ask yourself:
  - *Is my decision to delegate to this complementary therapy appropriate?* Evidence-based decisions are most persuasive; commonly accepted but unproven indications are also acceptable.
  - *Have I taken reasonable steps to ensure that the practitioner is qualified and insured?* Usually sufficient to ensure s/he is a member of the main professional regulatory body responsible for that discipline. Main bodies require members to be fully indemnified.
  - *Has my medical follow up been adequate?* Continue following up chronic conditions as usual. Don't issue repeat prescriptions without having sufficient information to ensure safe prescribing.
- *Referral to medically qualified practitioner/state registered osteopath or chiropractor:* Same legal situation as when referring to another conventional healthcare practitioner for any other service. As long as the decision to make the referral is appropriate (see above), all further responsibility is taken over by the practitioner providing the specialist service.

**Further information:**

Bandolier

⊟ www.jr2.ox.ac.uk/bandolier/booth/booths/altmed.html

# Acupuncture

Acupuncture means 'piercing with a sharp instrument'. Needles are used to alleviate symptoms or cure disease. Mechanism of action remains unclear. Broadly, two forms exist – traditional/Chinese and modern/Western. There is no 'right way' to practice as there are no scientific data comparing the two.

**Use and evidence:** Acupuncture has been used to treat all conditions but is commonly used in Europe and the USA to treat musculoskeletal problems and chronic disease. Although Table 6.1 reports the overall outcome of systematic reviews and good quality randomized controlled trials for various applications of acupuncture, it should be used with caution as there are very few large, good quality trials in existence and almost all are –ve.

## Contraindications:
- Unwilling or frightened patient
- Pregnancy (especially first trimester as anecdotal evidence suggests ↑ risk of miscarriage)
- Bleeding disorders and anticoagulant use (relative contraindication)
- Skin infections or diseased skin
- Disorders of the immune system
- Valvular heart disease (only if indwelling needles are used).

**Side effects:** Rare (1:1000 treatments) – include:
- Infection (ONLY go to practitioners using disposable needles)
- Bruising/haemorrhage
- Anatomical damage (pneumothorax most common)
- Needle fracture or needles left *in situ*
- Fainting
- Sweating
- Convulsions
- Miscarriage (anecdotal)

## Variants of acupuncture:

**Auriculotherapy:** Microsystem of acupuncture based on a 'homunculus' or map of the body on the ear. Stimulation of points on the ear representing an area in pain produces analgesia. Best known for treatment of addiction, especially smoking. No good quality evidence of effectiveness. Often practiced using semi-permanent needles in an attempt to prolong its effects at the risk of infection at the needle site. Should not be used for patients with artificial heart valves, valvular heart disease, or immune deficiency.

**Transcutaneous electrical nerve stimulation (TENS):** Electrodes are placed on the skin over the painful area or at other locations e.g. over cutaneous nerves, trigger points, acupuncture sites. The TENS unit passes electrical current through the electrodes. The patient can control strength of current and pulse interval. Widely used by midwives, physiotherapists and in hospitals. No good evidence of effectiveness.

**Reflexology:** A representation of the body is found on the foot. Diagnosis is through palpation of the sole of the foot for tender points. These correspond to the area of the body where there is pain. Treatment consists of massaging these points or applying acupressure to relieve symptoms. No good-quality evidence of effectiveness but unlikely to do any harm.

### Table 6.1 Evidence for common uses of acupuncture

| Largely positive | Inconclusive | Largely negative |
|---|---|---|
| Back pain[S] | Chronic pain[S] | Cocaine addiction[R] |
| Migraine[R] | Neck pain[S] | Smoking cessation[C] |
| Idiopathic headache[C] | Fibromyalgia[S]* | Stroke[S] |
| Osteoarthritis of the knee[R] | OA[S] | Carpal tunnel syndrome[C] |
| Postoperative nausea and vomiting (adults)[S] | RA[C] | Hot flushes[S] |
| | Tennis elbow[C] | Tinnitus[S] |
| | TMJ dysfunction[S] | |
| | Weight reduction[S] | |
| | Asthma[C] | |
| | Labour pain[C] | |

* Some evidence acupuncture caused exacerbation of symptoms for some patients

**Further reading:**
**Effective Health Care.** Acupuncture 2001 7(2)
🖳 www.york.ac.uk/inst/crd/ehcb.htm

### GP Notes: Professional organizations

**British Medical Acupuncture Society** ☎ 01925 730727; *Fax:* 01925 730492 🖳 www.medical-acupuncture.co.uk
**British Acupuncture Council** ☎ 020 8735 0400 🖳 www.acupuncture.org.uk
**Acupuncture Association of Chartered Physiotherapists** ☎ 01747 861151 *Fax:* 01747 861717 🖳 www.aacp.uk.com
**Association of Reflexologists** ☎ 0870 5673320 🖳 www.aor.org.uk
**British Homeopathic Library** 🖳 www.hom-inform.org

# Homeopathy

*From the Greek meaning 'treatment by similars'.*

**Theory of homeopathy:** Homeopathy works on the principle that 'like cures like'. The majority of homeopathic remedies are derived from plants although chemical and animal sources are also used. A remedy is chosen that mimics the symptoms displayed by the patient e.g. homeopathic ipecacuanha is used to treat nausea and vomiting. Most remedies are serially diluted in steps of 1:10 (decimal x) or 1:100 (centesimal c).

> ⚠ Some lay practitioners believe conventional drugs ↓ efficacy of homeopathy. It is important that users of homeopathic drugs do not stop taking conventional medicines unless advised to by the doctor who prescribed them.

**Use:** Often used to treat symptoms of acute self-limiting illness. Also used widely for chronic conditions e.g. eczema, stress, depression, and chronic fatigue. Homeopathic treatment is slow. The 'rule of 12' states 1mo. of treatment is required for each year the patient has the problem.

**Availability of drugs:** Manufacture of homeopathic medicine is controlled by the Medicines Act (1968). Homeopathic drugs can be purchased OTC at pharmacies and health food shops or prescribed on NHS prescription.

> ⚠ Legal responsibility for prescribing lies with the person who signs the prescription form.

**Side effects/contraindications:** Homeopathic remedies of sufficient dilution (>30x or 12c) and obtained from a reputable manufacturer are unlikely to cause adverse effects or interact with conventional medicines. Homeopathy also appears to be safe in women who are pregnant/breastfeeding but should not be used to treat serious conditions for which there is a proven conventional therapy.

**Evidence:** With higher dilutions (>12c), a theoretical problem arises as the solution may not contain any molecules of the mother substance. Nevertheless homeopaths claim more dilute solutions are *more effective*. A meta-analysis published in 1997 pooled all studies comparing homeopathy against placebo and concluded that, overall, homeopathy has some effect.[1] However, there is insufficient information about the use of homeopathy in most clinical situations to decide when and if homeopathy is a credible adjunct or alternative to conventional treatment.

1 Linde et al (1997). *Lancet* **350**: 834–43.

## Table 6.2 Evidence for common uses of homeopathy

| Largely positive | Inconclusive | Largely negative |
|---|---|---|
| Postoperative ileus[S] | Atopic eczema[S] | Bruising[S] |
| Dandruff and seborrhoeic dermatitis[R] | Chronic asthma[C] | Osteoarthritis[S] |
| | Ocular symptoms of hayfever[S] | Rheumatoid arthritis[S] |
| | Influenza[C] | Headache[S] |
| | Dementia[S] | Delayed-onset muscle soreness[C] |
| | Premenstrual syndrome[R] | Migraine prophylaxis[S] |
| | Low back pain[R] | |
| | Otitis media[R] | |
| | Acute sinusitis[R] | |
| | Labour pain[C] | |

### GP Notes: Professional organizations

**British Homoeopathic Association** ☎ 0870 444 3950
*Fax:* 0870 444 3960 🖳 www.trusthomeopathy.org
**Society of Homoeopaths** ☎ 01604 621400 *Fax:* 01604 622622
🖳 www.homeopathy-soh.org
**British Homeopathic Library** 🖳 www.hom-inform.org

# Herbal medicine

Use of plants or plant parts for medicinal purposes. Conventional medicine uses many drugs derived from herbal substances e.g. digoxin, aspirin, and morphine. Herbal medicine uses plant extracts, not isolated constituents. Herbalists believe different compounds contained in a herbal preparation act synergistically.

**Availability of herbal medicine:** Widely available in the UK. Most products are unlicensed and sold as foods. *Problems:*

- Quality assurance
- Accidental contamination
- Botanical quality
- Unknown optimum dose/dosage range
- Lack of data on drug interactions

⚠ Report all adverse herbal medicine reactions and drug interactions using the yellow card scheme. Keep a sample of the implicated herbal medicine.

**Uses and evidence:** Used for a wide range of conditions often with little evidence of efficacy. See Table 6.3.

**Aromatherapy:** Use of aromatic plant oils (usually by inhalation or application to the skin) for benefit. No good evidence of effectiveness. Oils used are extremely concentrated. *Uses:*

- Lavender oil — Burns, blisters, insomnia
- Tea tree oil — Headlice, athlete's foot, wound infection
- Geranium oil — Calming, antidepressant
- Eucalyptus oil — Clear blocked noses (Vicks Vaporub®)
- Thyme oil — Antiseptic – used for colds and flu
- Rosemary oil — Antiseptic and soothing – good for sinus infections
- Peppermint oil — Headache, indigestion
- Valerian oil — Anxiety and insomnia

**Cautions, side effects and contra-indications:** Volatile oils are readily absorbed through mucous membranes and may be as potent as any drug. Sold as unlicensed products – quality, safety, interactions and efficacy have not been assessed. Can be poisonous if ingested.

---

**GP Notes: Professional organizations**

**British Herbal Medical Association** ☎ 01202 433691
*Fax:* 01202 417079 🖥 www.bhma.info
**National Institute of Medical Herbalists** ☎ 01392 426022
*Fax:* 01392 498963 🖥 www.nimh.org.uk
**International Federation of Professional Aromatherapists**
☎ 01455 637987 🖥 www.ifparoma.org
**Aromatherapy Council** ☎ 0870 7743477
🖥 www.aromatherapycouncil.co.uk

## Table 6.3 Herbal products with evidence of efficacy

| Herb | Side effects | Evidence |
|------|-------------|----------|
| Saw Palmetto | Dizziness and mild GI effects. Rare: pruritus, headache, ↑BP. | BPH. Improvement in symptoms when used for >1–2 mo. Side effects < finasteride[C]. |
| Echinacea | Nausea, dizziness, SOB, dermatitis, pruritus and hepato-toxicity. Rare: allergy.<br>⚠ Advise patients NOT to take for >8wk. as can cause immune suppression. | Prevention and treatment of common cold – majority of studies +ve[C]. Theoretically may ↓ effects of immuno-suppressants and be harmful in autoimmune disease and HIV. |
| St. John's Wort | Dry mouth, GI symptoms, fatigue, headache, dizziness, skin rash, and ↑ sensitivity to sunlight.<br>Drug interactions: ↓ effect of anticonvulsants, warfarin, ciclosporin, digoxin, theophylline and COC pill.<br>Serotonergic effects (sweating, shivering, muscle contractions) with triptans and antidepressants.<br>⚠ DO NOT use concurrently with prescription antidepressants. | Depression – effective treatment. Discontinue 2wk. prior to surgery as theoretical risk of interaction with anaesthetic agents. |
| Gingko biloba | Spontaneous bleeding.<br>Drug interactions: ↑ effect of warfarin and antiplatelet agents. | Effective for improving cerebral blood flow[S] and intermittent claudication[S]. May help tinnitus[S]. |
| Feverfew | May cause breakthrough menstrual bleeding. Caution with anticoagulants. | Migraine prophylaxis – probably effective[C]. |
| Chinese herbal medicine | Serious blood dyscrasias and hepatotoxicity have been reported. | Effective for childhood eczema[S] and IBS[R]. |

### Other products for which there is evidence of effectiveness:
- Aloe vera (psoriasis[S] and genital herpes[S])
- Oil of evening primrose (RA[C])
- Kava (anxiety[S])
- Valerian (insomnia[S])
- Peppermint oil (IBS[S])
- Horse chestnut seed extract (chronic venous insufficiency[C])
- Yohimbine (erectile dysfunction[S])

### Further information:
Herbmed ⊠ www.herbmed.org

# Dietary manipulation and supplementation

*'Let your food be your medicine'*

Hippocrates (460–377 BC)

**Healing foods:** Branch of herbal medicine. Common examples for which there is some evidence of effectiveness include:

- *Chondroitin:* ↓ pain and symptoms of OA[S].
- *Cranberry juice:* Trial evidence for effect in prevention or treatment of UTI[R] not supported by Cochrane review[C].
- *Fish oil:* Cardioprotective effects[R]; ↓ pain and symptoms of RA[S].
- *Garlic:* ↓ cholesterol[S], antithrombotic/fibrinolytic effects[S] may have a role in cancer prevention.
- *Ginger:* ↓ nausea in a variety of situations[S].
- *Honey:* Wound dressing – improves healing[S].
- *Soya:* ↓ menopausal symptoms[S].
- *Yoghurt:* No evidence for treatment of vaginal infection or prevention of recurrence[S]. Mixed evidence[R] and no systematic reviews for treating diarrhoea with yoghurt.
- *Xylitol:* Some evidence *in vitro* and animal studies that ↓ bacterial infection. Currently under investigation for effects in minor illness e.g. sore throat.

**Nutritional medicine:** Involves prescribing vitamins, minerals, amino acids and essential fatty acids. Prescription is based on investigations into the individual's nutritional state by history taking, nutritional diaries and analysis of samples of blood, sweat and hair. Evidence of effectiveness:

- *Calcium supplements ± vitamin D:* ↓ incidence of osteoporosis and osteoporotic fracture[CS]. Calcium may ↓BP[S].
- *Folate supplements:* Taken preconceptually ↓ incidence of neural tube defect[R].
- *Glucosamine:* ↓ pain and symptoms of OA[C]. ⚠ Some products are derived from marine sources – patients allergic to shellfish should ensure product is synthetically manufactured.
- *Selenium:* Suggestion of protective effect against gastro-oesophageal cancer. No good-quality evidence and recent epidemiological data suggest supplements may be harmful.
- *Vitamin A:* Cancer prevention[S]. ⚠ Patients should NOT take supplements in pregnancy.
- *Vitamin B$_6$:* May be effective for premenstrual syndrome[S] but excessive ingestion (>2000mg/d.) causes peripheral neuropathy. Possible effect on autism[S].
- *Vitamin B$_{12}$:* No evidence of beneficial effect on cognition[C].
- *Vitamin C:* ↓ duration of symptoms of common cold if used in high doses[C]. May ↓ BP[S].
- *Vitamin E:* May have a role in prevention of cardiovascular disease[S]. Unclear whether helpful for dementia[C] and intermittent claudication[C].
- *Zinc:* Inconclusive evidence that it shortens duration of common cold[C].

**Probiotics:** Probiotics are orally administered microbial cell preparations or components of microbial cells that may have a beneficial effect on the health and well being of the host. There is some evidence of efficacy in treating a variety of medical problems including infectious diarrhoea[C], other gastrointestinal conditions including inflammatory bowel disease and irritable bowel syndrome, and atopy[S]. There is increasing interest in the use of probiotics in mainstream medicine and the evidence base for or against the use of these preparations is likely to increase over the next few years.

**Environmental medicine:** Based on the premise that individuals develop adverse responses to environmental substances, most commonly foods, which manifest as disease. Adverse reactions are termed 'allergies' or intolerance. This is a different use of the term allergy than that used in conventional medicine. In environmental medicine it means a reaction with insidious onset that is not predictable and does not trigger the immune pathways responsible for allergy.

Investigations involve diagnostic use of elimination diets or substance avoidance; challenge testing by exposure to the substance and the coca pulse test (speeding or slowing of the pulse by >10bpm after exposure).

🛈 Allergy testing machines based on electrical skin resistance are in common use although they produce inconsistent results and there is no evidence that they are predictive of intolerance.

Food intolerances are generally multiple with 1–2 'major' foods and several more 'minor' foods responsible for triggering effects. Common examples are: caffeine, milk, gluten, citrus fruit. Beware that patients on multiple exclusion diets do not become malnourished. There is very little evidence of effect – Cochrane review of use for recurrent childhood abdominal pain and systematic review of use for childhood eczema were both inconclusive.

---

**GP Notes: Professional organizations**

**British Herbal Medical Association** ☎ 01202 433691
🖥 www.bhma.info

# Physical therapies

**Osteopathy and chiropractic:** Physical treatments aimed at restoring alignment of the joints and improving functioning of the body. In the UK, both are distinguished from other complementary therapies by being under statutory regulation. All osteopaths and chiropractors have to undergo training lasting 4–5y. After that time, they are registered with their governing body which enforces a code of standards and discipline. They must have professional indemnity insurance.

**Osteopathy:** From Greek meaning 'bone disease'. Operates on the theory that if structure is improved, improvement in function follows.

**Chiropractic:** Diagnosis, treatment and management of conditions due to mechanical dysfunction of the joints and their effects on the nervous system. Chiropractors aim to restore normal alignment of joints.

**McTimoney chiropractic:** Branch of chiropractic that uses slightly different, gentler techniques than conventional chiropractic treatment.

**Method:** Osteopaths and chiropractors use standard orthopaedic techniques and may perform investigations including X-rays. They like to work closely alongside conventional physicians referring back to them any problems they detect outside their field of expertise. Treatment is usually physical using massage and joint manipulation. Both treat the whole patient, giving advice on posture, lifestyle, and prevention of musculoskeletal and other problems.

**Evidence:** Some good evidence of effectiveness especially for back pain[R].

**Massage:** 'If we hurt ourselves, we rub it better.' There are many different variants of massage, but the commonest seen in the UK are Swedish massage and Shiatsu or Japanese massage. Shiatsu uses a variant of acupressure (allied to acupuncture but using pressure on key points rather than needles) to enhance its effect.

**Evidence:** ↑ mobility[R], ↑ blood flow[R], ↑ expiratory volume[R] ↓ musculoskeletal and phantom limb pain[R], ↓ lymphoedema[R]. No convincing systematic review evidence of effect.

**Yoga:** Ancient art involving a sequence of physical stretches involving the whole body over a session. It is done slowly and in silence. Whilst performing the moves, participants breath slowly and deeply, fixing their minds on the activity they are doing. Yoga should be taught by an experienced instructor.

**Evidence:** ↓ seizure frequency for epileptics[C].

**Tai chi chuan:** Variously translated as 'supreme boxing' and the 'root of all motion'. It is considered a martial art but is not combative. It is based on fluidity and circular movements.

**Evidence:** ↓ falls and fear of falls in the elderly[R].

**Physiotherapy:** Physiotherapy is a health care profession concerned with maximizing potential, enhancing bodily function and preventing future problems. It uses mainly physical approaches to achieve this including:

- Manipulation
- Exercise
- Posture
- Massage
- Relaxation
- Ultrasound

Often, physiotherapists also use other complementary therapies during the course of their work e.g. acupuncture, aromatherapy, TENS.

Physiotherapists work in a wide variety of health settings and are widely used and appreciated by patients in the community for conditions ranging from stress, incontinence and chest disease to musculoskeletal problems. They are an integral part of the health care team and work closely with other members of the team.

**Evidence:** There is an extensive evidence base for the effectiveness of physiotherapy in a wide variety of conditions.

**Pilates:** Method of exercise involving physical movement designed to stretch, strengthen, and balance the body together with focused breathing patterns.

**Evidence:** No specific evidence though probably has the same benefits as general exercise.

---

**GP Notes: Professional organizations**

**General Osteopathic Council** ☎ 020 7357 6655
🖥 www.osteopathy.org.uk
**British Chiropractic Association** ☎ 0118 950 5950
🖥 www.chiropractic-uk.co.uk
**The Shiatsu Society** ☎ 0845 130 4560 🖥 www.shiatsusociety.org
**The British Wheel of Yoga** ☎ 01529 306 851 🖥 www.bwy.org.uk
**Tai Chi Union** ☎ 0141 810 3482 🖥 www.taichiunion.com
**Chartered Society of Physiotherapy** ☎ 020 7306 6666
🖥 www.csp.org.uk
**UK Pilates Foundation** ☎ 07071 781 859
🖥 www.pilatesfoundation.com
**Pilates Institute** ☎ 020 7253 3177 🖥 www.pilates-institute.com

# Counselling and cognitive behavioural therapy

**Counselling:** 1:3 problems brought to the GP have a psychosocial component. To cater for these patients most PCOs (81%) have some provision for practice-based counselling and 50% of practices have counselling services. Counselling services may also be available via community psychiatric or clinical psychology services.

## Table 6.4 Conditions suitable for referral to a counsellor

| Conditions suitable for referral for counselling | Conditions unsuitable for referral |
|---|---|
| Anxiety | Psychotic illness |
| Depression – especially minor depression | Phobias |
| Relationship problems | Obsessive–compulsive disorder |
| Bereavement | Eating disorder |
| After traumatic events | Personality disorder |
| Substance abuse | |

**Problem-solving therapy:** Another short-term therapy (typically 5–6 × 45min. sessions) which involves drawing up a list of problems, and generating and agreeing solutions, broken down into steps, for patients to work on as homework between sessions. Shown to be as effective as antidepressants for moderate depression[R].

## Cognitive behavioural therapy (CBT):

- *Behavioural therapies* aim to change behaviour. Usually the therapist uses a system of graded exposure (systematic desensitization) combined with teaching a method of anxiety reduction.
- *Cognitive therapy* focuses on peoples' thoughts and the reasoning behind their assumptions on the basis that incorrect assumptions → abnormal reactions which then reinforce these assumptions further (a vicious cycle).

## Table 6.5 Recognized professional bodies in the UK

**Counsellors**
- The British Association for Counselling and Psychotherapy (BACP)
- The UK Register of Counsellors
- The Association of Counsellors and Psychotherapists in Primary Care

**Psychologists**
- The British Psychological Society (chartered and counselling psychologists)

**Psychotherapists**
- The UK Council for Psychotherapy
- The British Confederation of Psychotherapists

## GP Notes: Frequently asked questions

**What is counselling?** There are no universally agreed definitions of the term 'counselling' or 'counsellor' and the distinction between counselling and psychotherapy is often unclear. Usually the key element in counselling is reflective listening to encourage patients to think about and try to resolve their own difficulties. It does not involve giving advice. Most counsellors use brief (time-limited) therapy offering patients a mean of 7 sessions each usually lasting ~50mins.

**Who is a counsellor?** There is no formal registration requirement in the UK for counsellors or psychotherapists. The GMC advises that GPs should only refer to practitioners who are members of a recognized disciplinary body and thus subject to ethical and disciplinary codes (Table 3.4).

**Does counselling work?** Many patients regard antidepressants as harmful or addictive and are increasingly reluctant to take them. They see counselling as an attractive alternative – a view supported by many GPs. Evidence shows counselling subjectively improves the condition the patient has been referred for and non-directive counselling is more effective than GP care in reducing anxiety and depression in the short term but not the long term. However, counselling does not ↓ drug costs and practices with counsellors make more referrals to 2° care psychiatric services. More research is needed into cost-effectiveness.

**Who should be referred?** Counsellors see a wide range of patients (Table 3.3). ~²/₃ of patients referred for counselling have significant levels of anxiety or depression.

**What is CBT used for?** CBT is of proven effectiveness in the treatment of mild depression, anxiety disorders, phobias, panic disorder, eating disorders and for the treatment of delusions and hallucinations in psychotic illness.

**How can patients be referred for CBT?** CBT is usually provided by highly trained psychotherapists and accessed via psychiatry services. Guided self-help programmes based on CBT are also effective for mild depression and can be delivered:
- Using books e.g. Gilbert. *Overcoming Depression*. Constable and Robin (2000). ISBN: 1841191256
- By computer e.g. *Beating the Blues*© (further information available from 🖥 www.ultrasis.com), or
- Via the Internet e.g. 🖥 www.psychologyonline.co.uk or The Mood Gym 🖥 www.moodgym.anu.edu.au

### Further information:

Psychol Med Bower et al. The clinical effectiveness of counselling in primary care (2003) **33**: 203–15

# Other complementary therapies

**Alexander technique:** Practical method for improving the way we 'use' ourselves in the activities of everyday life. No evidence of effectiveness but unlikely to be harmful.

**Art therapy:** Use of art as a therapeutic activity. Review of role in treatment of schizophrenia inconclusive[C].

**Autogenic training:** A type of relaxation technique which involves passive concentration and psychophysiological stimuli. There are six standard exercises to aid relaxation, ↑ warmth in the abdominal region and cool the cranial region. The technique takes ~8wk. to learn effectively and sessions 3x/d. are encouraged. It is used for a variety of conditions, including the treatment of hypertension. No evidence of effectiveness.

**Ayurveda:** Practised primarily in the Indian subcontinent for 5,000y. Ayurveda includes diet and herbal remedies and emphasizes the use of body, mind, and spirit in disease prevention and treatment. No good evidence of effectiveness.

**Faith healing:** Healing is an ancient art, practised by most civilisations, and given much prominence by the ancient Greeks. During the healing process, the healer transmits an 'energy' which produces a harmonizing and healing effect. This energy is transmitted in different ways according to the type of healer consulted. No good quality evidence of effect though one study did show prayer ↓ mortality in a cardiac unit[R].

**Hypnotherapy:** Hypnosis can be defined as a state of heightened suggestibility or altered state of consciousness where the subject feels very relaxed. In medical hypnotherapy, the patient is not controlled or manipulated and can normally remember what has taken place after the session has ended. Hypnotherapy consists of training the patient to relax very deeply – often with a focus, a scene, smell, touch sensation or colour, to aid this process. *Evidence:* No evidence of effectiveness for smoking cessation[C] or weight loss[C]. May be helpful for pain relief in labour[C] and to ↓ symptoms of IBS[S].

**Meditation:** The instructor gives each individual a phrase or word – the *mantra* – which must not be divulged. The process involves sitting quietly with eyes closed repeating the mantra for 20min. at a time 1–2x/d. The mantra focuses the mind on a single idea. If distractions occur they are observed and put out of mind. No good evidence of effectiveness.

**Reiki:** Japanese word representing 'universal life energy'. Reiki is based on the belief that when spiritual energy is channelled through a Reiki practitioner, the patient's spirit is healed, which in turn heals the physical body. No evidence of effectiveness.

**Relaxation:** Can either be carried out with a therapist or alone. A number of good relaxation tapes exist. It must be practised in a quiet environment.

- The patient starts in a comfortable position.
- S/he is asked to close his/her eyes and then focus on each part of the body in turn from toes upwards for a period of about 10sec. at each location.
- Often the patient is asked to feel the part of the body being focussed on becoming heavy.
- After this has been done, the patient is asked to visualize an idyllic scene, to breathe the smells, hear the sounds, and feel the textures.
- An image can be provided, such as a perfect evening on a warm, deserted beach.

Relaxation training is widely used throughout medicine. No convincing evidence of effect, but unlikely to be harmful.

---

**GP Notes: Professional organizations**

**Society of Teachers of the Alexander Technique** ☎ 020 7284 3338
🖳 www.stat.org.uk
**British Autogenic Society** ☎ 020 7383 5108
🖳 www.autogenic-therapy.org.uk
**National Federation of Spiritual Healers** ☎ 0845 1232777
🖳 www.nfsh.org.uk
**The Hypnotherapy Association** ☎ 01257 262124
🖳 www.thehypnotherapyassociation.org.co.uk
**UK Reiki Federation** ☎ 01264 773774 🖳 www.reikifed.co.uk

# Chapter 7

# Legal aspects of managing chronic pain and terminal illness in the community

# Controlled drugs (CDs)

**Writing prescriptions for CDs:** Any prescription for Schedule 2 and 3 controlled drugs (with the exception of temazepam) must contain the following details, written so as to be indelible:

- The patient's full name, address and age – if the patient is homeless, 'no fixed abode' is an acceptable address
- The patient's NHS (in Scotland, Community Health Index) number
- Name and form of the drug, even if only one form exists
- Strength of the preparation and dose to be taken
- The total quantity of the preparation, or the number of dose units, to be supplied in both words and figures e.g. 'Morphine sulphate 10 mg (ten milligram) tablets, one to be taken twice daily. Supply 60 (sixty) tablets, total 600 (six hundred) milligrams'
- Signature of the prescriber (must be handwritten) and date. It is good practice to include the GMC number of the prescriber as well.
- The address of the prescriber

!) Apart from in exceptional circumstances, prescriptions for CDs in Schedules 2,3 & 4 should be limited to a supply of ≤30d. treatment. The validity period of NHS and private prescriptions for Schedule 1, 2, 3 and 4 controlled drugs is restricted to 28 d. Schedule 2 and 3 drugs cannot be prescribed on repeat prescriptions or under repeat dispensing schemes.

**Controlled drugs register:** All health care professionals who hold personal stock of any Schedule 2 drugs must keep their own controlled drugs register, and they are personally responsible for keeping this accurate and up-to-date. Out-of-date drugs should be recorded and destroyed in the presence of an authorized witness (police, PCO official).

> **Prescriber's responsibilities**
>
> - To avoid creating dependence by unnecessarily introducing controlled drugs to patients.
> - Careful monitoring to ensure the patient does not gradually ↑ the dose of drug to a point where dependence becomes more likely.
> - To avoid being an unwitting source of supply for addicts. If you suspect an addict is attending surgeries with intent to obtain supplies, contact your PCO so that they can issue a warning to other practices.

**Misuse of Drugs Act (1971):** Controls manufacture, supply, and possession of controlled drugs. Penalties for offences are graded according to perceived harmfulness of the drug into three classes:

- *Class A:* e.g. cocaine, diamorphine (heroin), methadone, LSD, ecstasy.
- *Class B:* e.g. oral amphetamines, barbiturates.
- *Class C:* e.g. most benzodiazepines, androgenic and anabolic steroids, cannabis (recent downgrading).

**Misuse of Drugs Regulations (1985):** Defines persons authorized to supply and possess CDs while carrying out their professions and describes the way in which this is to be done. 5 schedules of drug:

- *Schedule 1:* Drugs not used for medicinal purposes e.g. LSD. Possession and supply prohibited except with special licence.
- *Schedule 2:* Drugs subject to full CD controls (written dispensing record, kept in locked container, CD prescription regulations) e.g. diamorphine, cocaine, pethidine.
- *Schedule 3:* Partial CD controls (as schedule 2 but no need to keep register – some drugs subject to safe custody regulations) e.g. barbiturates, temazepam, meprobamate, buprenorphine.
- *Schedules 4 and 5:* Most benzodiazepines, anabolic and androgenic steroids, HCG, growth hormone, codeine. Controlled drug prescription requirements do not apply nor do safe custody requirements.

**Further information:**

**National Prescribing Center (NPC)** A guide to good practice in the Management of controlled drugs in primary care (England) (2007) ⊟ www.npc.co.uk

---

**GP Notes: Travelling with controlled drugs**

🕕 For patients or doctors travelling abroad with schedule 2 or 3 drugs, an export licence may be required. Further details can be obtained from the Home Office (☎ 020 7273 3806). Patient applications must be accompanied by a doctor's letter giving details of:

- Patient's name and current address
- Quantities of drugs to be carried
- Strength and form of drugs
- Dates of travel

⚠ For clearance to import the drug into the country of destination, it is advisable to contact the Embassy or High Commission of that country prior to departure.

# Licensing of drugs

In the UK, the Medicines Act (1968) makes it essential for anyone who manufactures or markets a drug for which therapeutic claims are made, to hold a licence. The Licensing Authority, working through the Medicines and Healthcare Products Regulatory Agency (MHRA), can grant both Manufacturer's Licence and Marketing Authorization (which allows a company to market and supply a product for specified indications). Although doctors usually prescribe according to the licensed indications, they are not obliged to.

**Prescribing outside licence:** There may be occasions when a doctor feels it is necessary to prescribe outside a drug's licence:

- *Generic formulations* for which indications are not described. The prescriber has to assume the indications are the same as for branded formulations.
- *Use of well-established drugs for proven but not licensed indications* e.g. amitriptyline for neuropathic pain. Commonly occurs in palliative care (25% of prescriptions affecting 66% of patients) and chronic pain management. In most cases applies to 'new' uses for 'old' drugs where it is uneconomic for the manufacturer to obtain a licence.
- *Use of drugs for conditions where there are no other treatments* (even if the evidence of their effectiveness is not well proven). This often occurs in secondary care when new treatments become accepted. GPs may become involved if a patient is discharged to the community and the GP is asked to continue prescribing.
- *Use of drugs for individuals not covered by their licensed indications* frequently occurs in paediatrics.

> ⚠ Before prescribing any medication (whether within or outside the licence) weigh risks against benefits. The more dangerous the medicine, and the flimsier the evidence-base for treatment, the more difficult it is to justify the decision to prescribe.

### When prescribing licensed drugs for unlicensed indications:

- Inform patients and carers of what you are doing and why and obtain consent for the drug's use in that way.
- Explain that the patient information leaflet (PiL) will not have information about the use of the drug in these circumstances.
- Record in the patients notes your reasons for prescribing outside the licensed indications for the drug.

❶ The person signing the prescription is legally responsible.

**Use of established bodies of evidence:** If prescribing off-license, be able to justify your decision to use the drug in question. Established bodies of evidence can provide justification. Suitable sources include:

- Cochrane database
- Drugs and Therapeutics Bulletin
- British National Formulary
- Palliative Care Formulary
- Textbooks on palliative care and local palliative care guidelines

### Further information:

**DTB** Prescribing unlicensed drugs or using drugs for unlicensed applications (1992). **30:** 97–9

**European Journal of Anaesthesiology** Cohen P. Off-label use of prescription drugs: legal, clinical and policy considerations (1997). **14:** 231–50

**Association of Palliative Medicine and Pain Society.** The use of drugs beyond licence in palliaitive care and pain management (2002). www.britishpainsociety.org

**Twycross et al.** *Palliative Care Formulary 2.* (2002 2nd edition). Radcliffe Medical Press ISBN: 1857755111

**Palliative Drugs** ⊟ www.palliativedrugs.com

# Fitness to make decisions

**Definition:** *Mental capacity* is the ability to take actions affecting daily life (e.g. when to get up, what to wear, what to eat) and/or make more major decisions (e.g. where to live, how to manage money).

**Mental Capacity Act (2005):** came into force in 2007 in England and Wales. Similar legislation applies elsewhere in the UK. It specifies who can take decisions on behalf of other people and allows people to plan ahead for a time when they may lack capacity. 5 key principles:

- Every adult has the right to make decisions and must be assumed to have capacity to make them unless proved otherwise.
- Every adult must be given all possible help and support to make decisions, and to communicate those decisions where necessary, before s/he can be assumed to have lost capacity.
- Making an unwise decision does not mean that a person lacks capacity to make that decision.
- Anything done or any decision made on behalf of someone who lacks capacity must be done in his/her best interests.
- Anything done or any decision made on behalf of someone who lacks capacity should be the least restrictive of his/her basic rights/freedoms.

**Assessing capacity:** A GP asked to give an opinion on a patient's mental capacity, should:

- Have access to the patient's records and ideally know the patient
- Seek information from friends, relatives, carers and/or the patient's independent mental capacity advocate, if one has been appointed.
- Examine the patient, and assess the type and degree of deficit
- Decide if there is an impairment of, or disturbance in, the functioning of the patient's brain or mind
- If there is a disturbance, decide if the patient is able to make the particular decision in question – in particular: Can the patient understand the information relevant to that decision, including the likely consequences of making, or not making, that decision? Can the patient retain that information? Can the patient use or weight that information as part of the process of making the decision? Can the patient communicate that decision by any means?
- Decide if assessment should be postponed while measures are taken to improve capacity
- Record all the above information

⚠ Even if you think a proposed action is in the patient's best interests, you must not judge the patient capable if that is not clearly the case. If in doubt, seek a second opinion.

**Lasting Power of Attorney (LPA):** Replaced Enduring Power of Attorney (EPA) in October 2007. Patients with EPAs can still use them. An LPA is a legal document that lets individuals appoint someone they trust to make decisions for them. It can be drawn up at any time whilst the person has capacity, but has no legal standing until it is registered with the Office of the Public Guardian. 2 types:

- *Property and affairs LPA:* allows the 'attorney' to make decisions about management of money, property and affairs. Unless specified otherwise can be used even when the individual retains capacity.
- *Personal welfare LPA:* allows the 'attorney' to make decisions about healthcare and welfare, including decisions to refuse or consent to treatment and decide on place of residence. Only active when the LPA is registered and the individual lacks capacity to make decisions. The attorney can make decisions about life-sustaining treatment only if the LPA specifies that.

**Court of Protection:** If a person, by reason of mental disorder, becomes incapable of managing his or her affairs but has not previously signed an LPA, it may be necessary for someone, usually the nearest relative, to apply to the Court of Protection for the appointment of a 'receiver' to do so. The medical practitioner will be asked to complete form CP3. Alternatively, if the patient's affairs are simple (e.g. state pension) direct arrangements can be made with relevant authorities.

**Testamentary capacity:** The capacity to make a will. Anyone can make a will provided that they understand the nature and effect of making a will, extent of property being disposed of and claims others may have on that property, and the decision is not the result of their condition (e.g. due to a delusion)

🛈 Decisions don't have to seem rational to others, especially if consistent with pre-morbid personality.

**Advance decision:** statement about wishes regarding medical treatment in case the individual becomes incapable of making that decision later. Advance decisions are legally binding.

- Respect any refusal of treatment as long as the decision is clearly applicable to circumstances, there is no reason to believe the individual has altered that decision, and the decision was not made under duress
- Advance decisions do not have to be written, except those refusing life-sustaining treatment which must be: specific to a particular treatment (e.g. refusal to have CPR); written; signed by the person making the decision (or a representative if unable to sign), and a witness.
- Advance decisions cannot include decisions about treatment the person would like, only treatment the person refuses, and cannot include directions to end the person's life prematurely.
- Doctors may not be willing to carry through an advance directive. In such cases they should refer the patient to another doctor who is.
- The BMA recommends doctors should *not* withhold 'basic care' (e.g. symptom control) even in the face of a directive which specifies that the patient should receive no treatment.
- Where a formal advance statement is not available, take patients' known wishes into consideration.

### Further information:
Office of the Public Guardian 🖳 www.publicguardian.gov.uk
BMA local offices.
Medical defence organizations.

# Certifying fitness to work

**Own occupation test:** Applies to those claiming for the first 28wk. of their illness:
- statutory sick pay from their employer
- incapacity benefit who have done a substantial amount of work in the 21wk. prior to the illness.

The doctor assesses whether the patient is fit to do their *own* job.

**Personal capability assessment** *(formerly the 'All work test')*: Assesses a patient on a variety of different mental and physical health dimensions for ability to work. Not diagnosis dependant. Applies to:
- everyone after 28wk incapacity
- those who do not qualify for the own occupation test from the start of their incapacity.

Claimants are sent form IB50 to complete themselves and are asked to obtain form Med4 from their GP. If the Department of Work and Pensions (DWP) is not happy to continue paying their benefit on the basis of these reports, the applicant is called for a medical examination. Conditions which exempt patients from further examination are:
- Receipt of highest rate care component of disability living allowance (DLA), constant attendance allowance or >80% disabled for other benefit purposes
- Terminal illness
- Tetraplegia or paraplegia, hemiplegia, progressive neurological or muscle wasting disease
- Registered blindness
- Persistent vegetative state
- Severe mental illness or dementia
- Progressive immune deficiency (including AIDS)
- Severe learning disabilities
- Active and progressive polyarthropathy
- Severe progressive cardio-respiratory disease which persistently limits exercise tolerance.

**Private certificates:** Some employers request private certificates in the 1st week of sickness absence. They should request it in writing. If the GP chooses to provide the service, s/he may charge, both for a private consultation and the provision of a private certificate. The company should accept full responsibility for all fees incurred by the patient.

**Permitted work:** Incapacity benefits do allow very limited work – therapeutic work (must be done as part of a treatment programme and in an institution which provides sheltered work for people with disabilities); voluntary work; local authority councilor; disability expert on an appeal tribunal or member of the Disability Living Allowance advisory board (not >1d./wk.).

**Disability Discrimination Act 1995:** In some circumstances requires employers to make reasonable adjustments for an employee with a long term disability. Advise patients to seek specialist advice.

## Table 7.2 Forms for certifying incapacity to work

| | |
|---|---|
| SC1 | Self-certification form for people not eligible to claim Statutory Sick Pay who wish to claim incapacity benefit. |
| | Certifies first 7d. of illness. |
| | Available from local Jobcentre Plus offices and GP surgery. |
| SC2 | As SC1 but for people who can claim Statutory Sick Pay. |
| | Available from employer, local Jobcentre Plus offices and GP surgery. |
| Med 3 | Filled in by GP or hospital doctor who knows the patient for periods of incapacity to work likely to be >7d. |
| | If return within 14d. is forecast give fixed date of return ('closed certificate'). |
| | If longer, specify a period of time (e.g. 2mo.) ('open certificate'). Before the patient returns to work, reassess and give further certificate with fixed date of return. |
| | Only one Med 3 can be issued per patient per period of sickness. If mislaid, reissue and mark 'duplicate'. |
| Med 4 | See personal capability assessment (opposite). |
| | Only completed once for any period of incapacity from work. |
| Med 5 | Can be used if: |
| | • A doctor has not seen the patient but on the basis of a recent (<1mo.) written report from another doctor is satisfied that the patient should not work – the certificate should not cover a forward period of >1mo. |
| | • The patient returned to work without receiving a closed certificate (see Med 3 above). |
| | • >1d. since the patient was seen (so Med 3 or Med 4 cannot be issued) but it is clear that the disability is ongoing. |
| Med 6 | Used when it is felt that putting a diagnosis on a Med 3/Med 4 would be harmful either directly to a patient or through their employer knowing their diagnosis. |
| | A vague diagnosis is put on the form and a Med 6 completed which requests the Department for Works and Pensions (DWP) to send a form to obtain more precise details. |

### GP Notes: Useful information

**Department for Work and Pensions** Medical evidence for Statutory Sick Pay, Statutory Maternity Pay and Social Security Incapacity Benefit purposes: A guide for registered Medical Practitioners. IB204 (2004). 🖥 www.dwp.gov.uk

**Disability Discrimination Act** 🖥 www.direct.gov.uk/disability

# Fitness to drive

> ⚠ Driving licence holders (or applicants) have a legal duty to inform the DVLA of any disability likely to cause danger to the public if they were to drive. Insurance may become invalid if drivers do not inform their insurer of any change in medical circumstances.

**Driving licence types:**

- *Group 1* – Ordinary licence for driving a car/ motorcycle. Old licences expire at a person's 70th birthday and then must be renewed 3 yearly. Applicants are asked to confirm they have no medical disability. If so, no medical examination is necessary. New photocard licences are automatically renewed 10 yearly until age 70y. Minimum age 17y. (16y. if disabled).
- *Group 2* – Enable holders to drive lorries and buses. Min. age 21y. Initially valid until 45th birthday then renewable every 5y. until 65th birthday. >65y. renewable annually. Medical examination is needed to renew Group 2 licences. Applicants must bring form D4 (available from Post Offices) with them. Examinations take ~½h. A fee may be charged by the GP.

**Determining fitness to drive:** Patients with any disorder which may cause danger to others if they drove, should be advised not to drive and to contact the DVLA. The DVLA gives advice on when they can restart.

**Specific DVLA guidance regarding terminal illness:** Table 7.3

**Driving whilst taking drugs:** Doctors have a duty to inform patients when they are prescribed medication which may impair their driving (GMC guidelines). Many drugs used in patients with advanced disease may impair cognitive and motor skills including:

- Opioid analgesics
- Benzodiazepines e.g. diazepam, lorazepam
- Antidepressants e.g. amitriptyline
- Phenothiazines e.g. levomepromazine
- Antihistamines e.g. cyclizine

**Opioid analgesia:** Patients on long-term stable doses of opioids are permitted to drive. Patients starting opioids or after dose increase should be advised *not* to drive until fully adjusted to their new dose – usually takes 2–3wk.

**Seatbelt exemption:** Seatbelts prevent death and serious injury and it is compulsory for car occupants to wear seatbelts, where fitted. If patients cannot wear seatbelts e.g. due to a colostomy or extensive intra-abdominal disease, GPs can issue a seatbelt exemption form.

Certificates are available from the Department of Health, PO Box 777, London SE1 6XH; ☎ 08701 555455; Fax: 01623 724524; E-mail: doh@prologistics.co.uk

**Further information:**

DVLA. At a glance guide to the current medical standards of fitness to drive for medical practitioners 🖥 www.dvla.gov.uk

Medical advisers from the DVLA can advise on difficult issues – contact: Driver's Medical Unit, DVLA, Swansea SA99 1TU or ☎ 01792 761119

## Table 7.3 DVLA guidance about fitness to drive in terminal illness

| Condition | Group 1 licence restrictions | Group 2 licence restrictions |
|---|---|---|
| Brain tumour | Varies – consult DVLA | Varies – consult DVLA |
| Malignant tumour with high chance of cerebral metastasis | Notify DVLA if cerebral secondaries are present. | Contact DVLA – cases are considered on an individual basis. |
| Heart failure | Continue driving unless symptoms which distract the driver's attention. | Licence revoked if symptomatic.<br>Restored if symptoms are controlled following medical examination and exercise ECG as long as left ventricular ejection fraction is >0.4. |
| Chronic neurological disease e.g. MS, Parkinson's disease, MND | Can be licensed if medical assessment confirms driving performance is not impaired – but a short period licence may be required.<br>If the driver requires a restriction to certain controls, this must be specified on the licence. | If condition is progressive or disabling – revoked.<br>If stable and driving is not impaired, can be considered for licensing subject to satisfactory medical report and annual review. |
| HIV/AIDS | Continue driving unless associated disability likely to affect driving. | Cases are assessed on an individual basis. In the absence of symptoms, CD4 count must be maintained at ≥200 for ≥6mo. to be eligible. |

### GP Notes: What should I do if a patient continues to drive despite advice to stop?

**If the patient _does not_ understand the advice to stop driving:** Inform the DVLA.

**If the patient _does_ understand the advice to stop driving:**

- Explain your legal duty to breach confidentiality and inform the DVLA if they do not stop driving.
- If the patient still refuses to stop driving, offer a second medical opinion – on the understanding that they stop driving in the interim.
- If the patient still continues driving, consider action such as recruiting next-of-kin to the cause – but beware of breach of confidentiality.
- If all else fails, write to the patient to inform him/her of your intention to inform the DVLA.
- If the patient continues to drive, inform the DVLA and write to the patient to confirm a disclosure has been made.

🔸 Always consider contacting your medical defence body for advice.

# Fitness to fly and perform other activities

**Fitness to fly:** Passengers are required to tell the airline at the time of booking about any conditions that might compromise their fitness to fly. The airline's medical officer must then decide whether to carry them.

*Hazards of flying:*
- Cabin pressure – oxygen levels are lower than at ground level and gas in body cavities expands 30% in flight
- Inactivity and dehydration
- Disruption of routine
- Alcohol consumption
- Stress and excitement

**Fitness to perform sporting activities:** GPs are commonly asked to certify fitness to perform sports. Normally the patient will come with a medical form. If there is a form, request to see it before the medical. If there is no form and you are unsure what to check, telephone the sport's governing body or the event organizer. A fee is payable by the patient.

Many gyms and sports clubs also ask older patients and patients with pre-existing conditions or disabilities to check with their GP before they will sign them on. Assuming that a suitable regime is undertaken, most people can participate in some form of sporting activity. Consider the patient's baseline fitness, check BP and medications and recommend a gradual introduction to any new forms of exercise.

**Pre-employment certification:** It is becoming increasingly common for GPs to be asked about the 'medical' suitability of candidates to perform a job. This is not part of the GP's terms of service and therefore a GP can refuse to give an opinion. In all cases where an opinion is given, a fee can be claimed. Common examples are:
- Ofsted forms for childminders
- Care home staff – proof of 'physical and mental fitness'
- Food handlers – certificates of fitness

## GP Notes

⚠ Remember – signing a form may result in legal action against you should the patient NOT be fit to undertake an activity.

Where possible include a caveat e.g. 'based on information available in the medical notes the patient appears to be fit to … although it is impossible to guarantee this.'

If unsure, consult your local LMC or medical defence organization for advice.

# Confirmation and certification of death

> ⚠ The death certification process in England and Wales is currently under review and likely to change in the near future.

English law *does not* require a doctor:
- To confirm death has occurred or that 'life is extinct'. A doctor is only required to certify what, in their opinion, was the cause.
- To view the body of a deceased person. There is no obligation to see/examine a body before issuing a death certificate.
- To report the fact that death has occurred.

English law *does* require the doctor who attended the deceased during the last illness to issue a certificate detailing the cause of death. Certificates are provided by the local Registrar of births, marriages and deaths. A special certificate is needed for infants of <28d. old.

**Death in the community:** ¼ occur at home.

**Expected deaths:** In all cases, advise to contact the undertakers and ensure the patient's own GP is notified.
- *Patient's home:* visit as soon as practicable.
- *Residential/nursing home:* if possible, the GP who attended during the patient's last illness should visit and issue a death certificate. The 'on-call' GP is often requested to visit. There is no statutory duty to do this but it is reassuring for the staff at the home and often necessary before staff are allowed to ask for the body to be removed.

**Unexpected and/or 'sudden' death:** If called, advise the attendant to call the emergency services. Visit and take a rapid history from any attendants. Then:
- *Resuscitate if appropriate* – Drowning and hypothermia can protect against hypoxic neurological damage; brains of children <5y. old are more resistant to damage.
- *Report the death to the coroner* – If any suspicious circumstances or circumstances of death are unknown/unclear, call the police.

*Alternatively*, if police or ambulance service is already in attendance and death has been confirmed, suggest the police surgeon is contacted.

**Cremation:** The Cremation Regulations (2008) require 2 doctors to complete a certificate to establish identity and that the cause of death is not suspicious before a person can be cremated. The person arranging the funeral may see the forms and pays a fee to each doctor. There are 2 parts:
- *Cremation 4* Completed by the patient's usual medical attendant – usually his/her GP.
- *Cremation 5* Completed by another doctor who must have held GMC registration (or equivalent) for ≥ 5y. and is not connected with the patient in any way nor directly connected with the doctor who issued cremation form 4 – usually a GP from another practice.

> ⚠ Pacemakers and radioactive implants must be removed from the deceased before cremation can take place.

> ### Box 7.1 Deaths which must be reported to the coroner
>
> - Sudden or unexpected deaths
> - Accidents and injuries
> - Industrial diseases e.g. mesothelioma
> - Service disability pensioners
> - Deaths where the doctor has not attended within the past 14d.
> - Deaths arising from ill treatment e.g. abuse, neglect, starvation, hypothermia
> - Cause of death unknown
> - Deaths <24h. after hospital admission
> - Poisoning (chronic alcoholism and its sequelae are no longer notifiable)
> - Medical mishaps (including anaesthetic complications, short- or long-term complications of operations, drugs – whether therapeutic or addictive)
> - Abortions
> - Prisoners
> - Stillbirths (if there is doubt about whether the baby was born alive)
> - CJD

**Notification of death to the coroner:** The coroner can be contacted via the local police. Reporting to the coroner does not automatically entail a post mortem. The coroner, once circumstances of death are clear, may advise the GP to tick and initial box A on the back of the certificate which advises the Registrar that no inquest is necessary. Deaths which *MUST* be reported to the coroner are listed in box 7.1.

ⓘ In Scotland, deaths are reported to a procurator fiscal. The list of reportable deaths is the same with the addition of deaths of foster children and the newborn.

**Recording deaths at the practice:** Death registers are useful. Routine communication of deaths to all members of the primary healthcare team and other agencies involved with the care of that patient (e.g. hospital consultants, social services) avoids the embarrassing and distressing situation of ongoing appointments and contacts being made for that patient. Record the death in the notes of any relatives/partner registered with the practice.

### Benefits available after a death

- For widows/widowers: 📖 pp.240–1
- Funeral payment: 📖 p.244

> ### Advice for patients
>
> #### Department of Work and Pensions (DWP)
> - Leaflet D49: What to do after a death in England and Wales. Available from 🖥 www.dwp.gov.uk/publications/dwp/2006/d49_april06.pdf
> - Funeral payment: Information and online application from 🖥 www.jobcentreplus.gov.uk
>
> **Scottish Executive.** What to do after a death in Scotland. Available from 🖥 www.scotland.gov.uk/library5/social/waad-00.asp

# Organ donation

>5,500 people in the UK are waiting for an organ transplant that could save or dramatically improve their life but <3,000 transplants are carried out each year. There is a desperate need for more donors. In 2003, ~400 people died while waiting for a transplant.

## Absolute contraindications to any organ donation:

- Untreated systemic infection
- HIV
- Hepatitis B or C
- Alzheimer's disease and other diseases of unknown aetiology (e.g. MS, MND)
- Creutzfeld-Jacob disease
- Any high-risk factor for HIV (defined by DoH as: homosexual men, prostitutes, history of IV drug abuse, haemophiliacs, people who have had sexual relations with local people from Africa south of the Sahara since 1977, sexual partners of people in these groups)

**Donor cards and the NHS Organ Donor Register:** Potential donors should always discuss their wishes with their relatives. They can register their desire to donate their organs after death by adding their names to the NHS Organ Donor Register and/or obtaining an Organ Donor Card. Contact the NHS Organ Donor Line ☎ 0845 60 60 400 or sign up online at 🖥 www.uktransplant.org.uk

**Live donation:** Certain tissues can be donated whilst a donor is alive:
- *Blood:* Contact the Blood Transfusion Service ☎ 0845 7 711 711 🖥 www.blood.co.uk (in South, Mid, East and West Wales ☎ 0800 25 22 66 🖥 www.welshblood.org.uk). New donors age 17–59y. are accepted and donors can continue giving blood until aged 70y.
- *Bone marrow:* Contact the British Bone Marrow Registry ☎ 0845 7 711 711 🖥 www.blood.co.uk (in South, Mid, East and West Wales contact the Welsh Bone Marrow Registry ☎ 0800 371 502 🖥 www.welshblood.org.uk). A blood sample is taken on registration to allow tissue matching. Donation involves a small operation in which bone marrow is harvested – usually from iliac crests.
- *1 kidney, part of lung, liver or small intestine:* usually close relatives. Removal of the organ/part-organ involves a major operation for the donor. Risks to donor must be weighed vs. benefits to recipient.

## Donation after death: Table 7.4
- *Heart-beating donation:* Donors must be maintained on a life-support machine at the time of death and until the organs are removed. The role of the GP in these situations is pre-emptive (information about organ donor register/donor cards) and to support families to make the decision whether to donate. Organs that can be donated are the kidneys, heart, liver, lungs, pancreas, corneas, heart valves, bone and skin.

- **Non-heart-beating donation:** The most important group for GPs as donation can occur even if the patient dies in the community. The GP must initiate removal of tissues by contacting the local organ transplant co-ordinator or the National Blood Services Tissue Services Division ☎ 07693 086823.
- **Donation of whole body for medical education:** Contact HM inspector of Anatomy (☎ 020 7972 4342/4551). Relatives should contact the medical school with which the donor has made arrangements after their death. Medical schools arrange collection of the body and a simple funeral. Not all bodies are accepted. The donor *must* give authorization for donation prior to death.
- **Tissue donation after death for research purposes:** Can be done in addition to donation for transplantation – organs for transplant are taken first 🖥 www.bodydonation.org.uk

**Approach to relatives:** Many families find the act of donation a source of comfort. Even with a signed donor card, the relatives of the patient must give their consent to organ donation post mortem.

**The Coroner:** For any patient normally referred to the Coroner, the Coroner's permission must be gained before tissues are removed.

**Further information:**

United Kingdom Transplant 🖥 www.uktransplant.org.uk

| Table 7.4 Organs suitable for non-heart-beating donation | | |
|---|---|---|
| Organ | Criteria for donation | Specific contraindications |
| Corneas | >1y. old. No upper age limit. May be retrieved up to 24h. after death. | Scarring/ulceration of cornea Leukaemia/certain lymphomas Malignancy otherwise is *not* a contraindication, neither is poor eye sight. |
| Heart valves | 3mo.–60y. May be retrieved up to 48h. after death. | Congenital valve defect Rheumatic heart disease Cardiac arrest/MI and malignancy are *not* contraindications. |
| Skin | 16–85y. >1.7m tall and >70kg weight. May be retrieved up to 48h. after death. | Prolonged steroid therapy Chronic skin disease e.g. psoriasis Malignancy |
| Bone | ≥16y. No upper age limit. May be retrieved up to 24h. after death. | Any history of malignancy Osteomyelitis RA Traumatic bone fractures |

# Euthanasia

The word Euthanasia originates from the Greek 'eu' meaning 'good' and 'thanatos' meaning 'death'. It usually means a deliberate intervention undertaken with the express intention of ending a life so as to relieve intractable suffering, performed at request of the person who will die or with their consent. However, some people define euthanasia to include both voluntary and involuntary termination of life.

**Involuntary euthanasia:** Killing of a person who has not explicitly requested aid in dying. This is most often done to patients who are in a persistent vegetative state and will probably never recover consciousness. It is not a decision that a GP would ever have to make and is therefore beyond the scope of this text.

**Passive euthanasia:** Hastening the death of a person by altering some form of support and letting nature take its course. Examples include:

• Turning off life support equipment for patients who are 'brain dead'.
• Withdrawing medical procedures or treatments.
• Stopping food and/or water.
• Not delivering CPR if the patient has a cardiac or respiratory arrest.
• The 'dual' or 'double' effect in which patients are given large doses of opioid analgesics to remove pain, at the cost of respiratory depression and hastening of death (□ p.88).

In most societies 'passive euthanasia' is acceptable for very elderly or frail patients or those with terminal illness, so that a death which was approaching comes sooner – though it is advisable to discuss any measures which may hasten death with the patient (if possible) and all close family members. If in doubt, consult your medical defence body.

Where there is disagreement between family/patient and medical attendants, recourse to the courts is sometimes necessary.

### Active euthanasia and physician-assisted suicide:

• Active euthanasia is death of a person through a direct action, in response to a request from that person.
• In physician-assisted suicide or voluntary passive euthanasia, a physician supplies information and/or the means of committing suicide (e.g. a prescription for lethal dose of sleeping pills) to a patient so that s/he can easily terminate his/her own life.

❶ The American State of Oregon, the Netherlands and Belgium are the only jurisdictions in the world where laws specifically permit euthanasia or assisted suicide. Oregon permits assisted suicide; the Netherlands and Belgium permit both euthanasia and assisted suicide. Both are illegal in the UK.

### Reasons why patients want to end their lives:

• *Depression:* 'A permanent solution to a temporary problem.' There is consensus that depression should never be a reason for euthanasia – treatment is a better solution.

- *Excessive pain:* This is a common reason cited for euthanasia but usually reflects inadequate clinical care. Better analgesia can give patients considerable amounts of good quality life – even if overall prognosis is poor.
- *Poor quality of life/loss of dignity* – the patient has a disease which severely affects quality of life and/or dignity to the point that the patient no longer wants to live that way. Alternatively, the patient may have been diagnosed with a progressive disease which will result in a decreasing quality of life/dignity and would rather die before quality of life/dignity is lost e.g. MND, Huntington's chorea.
- *Need for control:* The patient knows s/he will die in the near future and wants control over that process with suicide as an option. In a study done in Oregon looking at the first year of legalization of physician-assisted suicide, at least 6 of the 23 patients who obtained medication to end their lives did not use it and actually died a natural death.

**The ethical debate:** The subject of voluntary euthanasia is far from simple – even the most sympathetic cases raise difficult ethical questions.

### Arguments for euthanasia:
- It is a matter of personal freedom – human beings have the right to decide when and how to die.
- As suicide is no longer a crime in the UK, supporters of euthanasia argue that it is not only just, but also an essential part of civilization that people can be helped to die in dignity and pain free.
- Refusing to help someone when suffering intolerable pain or distress is immoral. It could even cause more injury and distress if the suicide attempt is botched.
- Euthanasia happens anyway – it is better to have it out in the open so that it can be properly regulated and carried out.
- There is no difference between withdrawing life sustaining therapy and actively ending life – in fact, withdrawing life sustaining therapy may be a cruel option resulting in a more prolonged and uncomfortable death.

### Arguments against euthanasia:
- Some religious groups believe life is sacrosant and only God can decide when to terminate it. They argue that we suffer for a reason.
- Others believe euthanasia weakens society's belief in the sanctity of life.
- Voluntary euthanasia is the start of a slippery slope – allowing any system of legalized killing would be open to abuse and lead to patients being pushed into agreeing to euthanasia, involuntary euthanasia and killing to save money or remove 'undesirables' from society.
- Proper palliative care reduces the need for euthanasia and allowing euthanasia may lead to less good care for the terminally ill.
- There is no sure way of controlling euthanasia.
- It is dangerous to make a universal law on the basis of a minority of particular cases.

It is beyond the scope of this text to come to any ethical conclusions or take any stance on the debate over euthanasia.

### Further information:
**BBC** Balanced information about the euthanasia debate and links to other sites ⊞ www.bbc.co.uk/religion/ethics/euthanasia

# Benefits and support available for people with chronic pain and terminal illness and their carers

# Benefits

> ⚠ Information in this section is up to date at the time of going to press but benefits issues change rapidly.

Millions of pounds of benefits go unclaimed every year. This chapter is a rough guide to the benefits available to enable GPs to point their patients in the right direction. It is not intended as a comprehensive reference.

**Table 8.1 Guide to agencies involved in delivering benefits to patients**

| Agency | Function | Website: http://www. + suffix | Telephone |
|---|---|---|---|
| Department for Work and Pensions (DWP) | Administers all benefits *except:* Tax credits (Inland Revenue) Statutory Sick Pay (employer) Housing Benefit (local authority) Council tax benefit (local authorities) | dwp.gov.uk | *Benefits Enquiry Line –* 0800 882200 *Help with form completion –* 0800 441144 *Information for employers and the self-employed –* 0845 7143143 |
| Jobcentre Plus | Helps people of working age to find work and get any benefits they are entitled to | jobcentreplus. gov.uk | Contact local office (list available on website) |
| Pension Service | Provides services and support for pension- ers and people looking into pensions and retirement | thepensionservice. gov.uk | Contact area office (list available on website) |
| HM Reve- nue and Customs | Administers tax credits | hmrc.gov.uk | Tax credit enquiry line – 0845 300 3900 |
| Disability and Carers Service | Delivers a range of benefits to disabled people and their carers | direct.gov.uk/ disability | N/A |
| Tribunals Service | Provides an independent tribunal body for hearing appeals | appeals-service. gov.uk | N/A |

🛈 0800 numbers are free; 0845 numbers are charged at local rate.

⚠ Benefit fraud: The DWP provides a freephone number which members of the public can telephone in confidence to give information about benefit fraud. ☎ 0800 85 44 40

**Further information for health professionals:**
Department for Work and Pensions (DWP)
🖥 www.dwp.gov.uk

**Further information for patients and carers:**
Government Information and Services 🖥 www.direct.gov.uk
Citizens Advice Bureau 🖥 www.adviceguide.org.uk
Age Concern ☎ 0800 00 99 66 🖥 www.ageconcern.org.uk
Counsel and Care ☎ 0845 300 7585 🖥 www.counselandcare.org.uk

# Pensions and bereavement benefits

**War pensions:** For people injured whilst serving in the armed forces and their dependants (if injury caused or hastened death). Administered by the Veterans Agency, Ministry of Defence. No time limit for claims. *Benefits:*

**War pensions scheme:** for ex-Service personnel whose injuries, wounds and illnesses arose prior to 6$^{th}$ April 2005.

### War Disablement Pension:
- *Basic benefits:* based on percentage disablement
  - If <20% disabled – lump sum
  - If >20% disabled – weekly sum (pension)
- *Other benefits:* Allowances if severely disabled e.g.:
  - War Pensioners mobility supplement – for walking difficulty. Holders can apply for the motability scheme and road tax exemption .
  - Constant attendance allowance – for high levels of care.

*Medical treatment:* Some services and appliances may be paid for by the Veterans Agency (includes prescription charges, nursing home fees)

*War Widows and widowers' pensions:* for spouses/civil partners of Service/ex-Service personnel:
- Where death was a result of Service or
- If the deceased was in receipt of a War Pensions Constant Attendance Allowance.
- If the deceased was in receipt of a War Disablement Pension at the rate of ≥80% and was getting Unemployability supplement

*War widow's and widower's allowances:* automatic age allowance when widows/widowers reach 65y. and further increase at 70y. and 80y.

**Armed Forces Compensation Scheme (AFCS):** provides benefits for illness, injury or death caused by service on or after 6$^{th}$ April 2005. Time limit is 5y. from the event, from the time when medical advice was first sought or after retirement – whichever is soonest. There is an exceptions list for late onset conditions. Provides:
- Lump sum for significant illnesses/injuries – 15 levels of award
- Tax-free Guaranteed Income Payment (GIP) for life for injuries at the higher tariff levels (1-11) to compensate for loss of earnings capacity
- Guaranteed Income Payment for Survivor's (SGIP) where an attributable death occurs

**Retirement pension:** A state retirement pension is currently payable to women aged ≥ 60 y. and men aged ≥65 y. – even if still working. Entitlement age will rise to 65y. for women between 2010 and 2020 (affects those born April 1950 to April 1955). Claim forms should be received automatically – if not request one through the local Jobseeker Plus office. Pensions are taxable.

*Basic pension:* Flat rate amount – different for single people and married couples. If not enough National Insurance (NI) contributions have been paid, amounts may d. >80y. a higher rate is payable which is not dependant on NI contributions.

*Increase for dependants:* Paid if:
- The claimant's spouse is <60y. and earns under a set amount / does not receive certain other benefits
- The claimant has children (if claim made before April 2003).

*Additional pension:* State second pension (replaced SERPS). Based on NI contributions and earnings. Workers can opt out of the additional pension scheme, pay into a private or company scheme instead and pay lower NI.

*Graduated pension:* Some people may be entitled to a graduated pension. This is based on earnings between 1961 and 1975.

*Extra pension:* For a person who defers claiming retirement pension for up to 5 y.. Extra pension is payable when retirement pension is claimed.

0 If hospitalized, retirement pension is payable for 1y. at full rate. After 12 mo., basic pension is d but additional pension stays the same.

### Other benefits for pensioners:
- *Free colour TV license:* All pensioners > 75y.
- *Winter fuel payment:* Annual payment to all pensioners >60y.

**Home Responsibilities Protection (HRP):** Scheme which protects Basic State Pension for people who don't work or have low income and are caring for someone. 🖳 www.thepensionservice.gov.uk

**Christmas bonus:** One-off payment made to people receiving a retirement pension or income support a few weeks before Christmas.

**Bereavement benefits:** Payable to men and women whose spouses have died – including civil partnership but co-habitation does not qualify except in Scotland. Claims can be made on forms available from Benefits offices or on-line via 🖳 www.jobcentreplus.gov.uk. *Benefits available:*

**Bereavement payment:** Lump sum payable if spouse has paid enough National Insurance contributions, or death was caused by employment, and the recipient is below state pension age at the time of the death. Claim <12mo. after death.

**Widowed parent's allowance:** Paid to widows/widowers with children or if pregnant.

**Bereavement allowance:** Paid for 52wk. from the date of bereavement for spouses >45y. old, not bringing up children and under retirement age.

### Other benefitsfor widows/widowers:
- *Funeral payment* – 📖 p. 244
- *War Widows/widowers* – ☎ 0800 169 22 77 🖳 www.veterans-uk.info

### Further information:
**The Pension Service** 🖳 www.thepensionservice.gov.uk
**Pensions Advisory Service (TPA)** ☎ 0845 601 2923 🖳 www.pensionsadvisoryservice.org.uk
**Citizens Advice Bureau** 🖳 www.adviceguide.org.uk
**Veterans Agency** ☎ 0800 169 22 77 🖳 www.veterans-uk.info

## Table 8.2 Benefits for people with low income

| | Eligibility | How to apply | Benefits gained |
|---|---|---|---|
| Income Support (IS) | • ≥18y. (16y. in some circumstances) and <60y.<br>• Low income, <£8000 in savings (£16000 if in residential care) and not in receipt of JSA<br>• <16h. paid work/wk. (and partner <24h./wk.) | Form A1 from local Jobcentre Plus office | *Money* – depends on circumstances<br>*Other benefits* – housing benefit, community tax benefit, health benefits, and social fund payments. Children <5y. and pregnant women – free milk and vitamins. Children >5y. – free school meals and, in some areas, uniform grants.<br>*Christmas bonus* – 📖 p.241 |
| JobSeekers Allowance (JSA) | • ≥19y. and <60y. (women) or <65y. (men)<br>• Unemployed or working <16h./wk.<br>• Capable of and available for work<br>• Have a JobSeekers agreement that contracts the recipient to actively seek work | Apply by visiting local Jobcentre | *Contributions-based JSA* – can claim for up to 26wk. Age-dependent fixed weekly payment.<br>*Income-based JSA* – allowance dependent on circumstances. Entitles claimants to same benefits as income support (see above).<br>*Hardship payments* – available to people disallowed JSA. |
| Pension credit | *Guarantee credit* – ≥60y. and income below the appropriate amount. Appropriate amount varies according to circumstances. Capital (excluding value of own home) >£6000 is deemed to count as income at the rate of £1/wk./£500 capital.<br>*Savings credit* – ≥65y. and income > savings credit starting point – currently >£114.05/wk. for a single person or >£174.05 if one of a couple. Depends on level of income and circumstances. | Apply on form PC1<br>☎ 0800 991234 | *Money* – depends on circumstances<br>*Other benefits* – if receiving guarantee credit: automatically eligible for housing benefit, community tax benefit, and social fund payments. |

| | | |
|---|---|---|
| Working tax credit (WTC) | • Age ≥16y., working ≥16h./wk. and responsible for a child (<16y. or 16-19y.) in full-time education) <br> • Age ≥16y., working ≥16h./wk. and has a disability <br> • Age ≥50y., working ≥16h./wk. and has started work after ≥6mo. of receiving 1 of certain benefits. <br> • Age ≥25y. and working ≥30h./wk. | Apply to Inland Revenue <br> ☎ 0845 300 3900 <br> 🖳 www.hmrc.gov.uk | **Tax credits** – depends on adding together elements <br> • Basic element – paid to everyone entitled to WTC <br> • Second adult element <br> • Lone parent element <br> • Working >30h./wk. (can combine both parents if have children). <br> • Disability (if working >16h./wk.) <br> • Severe disability (if working >16h./wk.) <br> • Aged ≥50y. and in receipt of certain benefits before resuming work <br> • Childcare – up to 70% childcare costs |
| Children's tax credit (CTC) | • Age ≥16y. and <br> • Responsible for ≥1 child (<16y. or 16-19y. and in full time education). <br> • Family income <£50,000 pa. | Apply to Inland Revenue <br> ☎ 0845 300 3900 <br> 🖳 www.hmrc.gov.uk | **Tax credits** <br> • Family element – credit for any family eligible – if there is a child <1y. old in the family. <br> • Child element – credit for each individual child in the family – if the child is disabled/severely disabled. |
| Health benefits | **Automatic entitlement** <br> • Age >60y. or <16y. (19y. if in full time education) <br> • Claiming IS or income-based JSA <br> • Pregnant or within 1y. of child birth <br> **By application** <br> • Low income and <br> • Savings <£8000 | If automatic exemption, no need to claim. If not, claim using form HC1 available from pharmacies, GP surgeries and local Jobcentre Plus offices. | **Free** <br> • Prescriptions <br> • NHS dentistry <br> • NHS eye tests and glasses <br> • NHS wigs and fabric supports <br> • Travel to hospital <br> • Milk and vitamins for pregnant and breast-feeding women, and children <5y. |

| | Eligibility | How to apply | Benefits gained |
|---|---|---|---|
| Housing benefit | Low income, living in rented housing.<br>*Exclusions:* Full time students without dependants, people in residential care or with savings >£16,000. | Via local authority | Pays rent for up to 60wk. Then need to reapply. |
| Council tax benefit and second adult rebate | • **Council tax benefit:** Low income. Exclusions as for housing benefit.<br>• **Second adult rebate:** Payable if someone who lives with you is aged >18y, does not pay rent or council tax and has low income.<br>• **Council tax reduction:** If single occupier or disabled.<br>• **Disregarded occupants:** Certain people including students, carers and children, are not counted in calculating the number of people living at a property. | Via local authority | **Council tax benefit:** pays council tax<br>**Council tax reductions**<br>• Single occupier – 25% discount<br>• All disregarded occupants – 50%<br>• Disabled – reduction to next lowest council tax band |
| The 6 Social Fund payments | • **Crisis loan** – anyone except students and people in residential care can apply.<br>• **Budgeting loan** – for large purchases. Must receive IS, pension credit or income-based JSA.<br>• **Funeral payments** – Must receive low income benefit and be responsible for the funeral.<br>• **Cold weather payments** – average temperature <0°C for ≥7d. Must receive IS, pension credit or income-based JSA and live with a pensioner, child <5y. or disabled person.<br>• **Maternity grant**<br>• **Community care grant** – 📖 p.245 | Cold weather payments – should be automatic.<br>All others claim via local Jobcentre Plus offices or 🖥 www.jobcentreplus.gov.uk | • **Crisis loan** – up to £1000 – interest-free loan repayable when crisis finished over 78wk.<br>• **Budgeting loan** – as crisis loan<br>• **Funeral expenses** – sum towards cost of funeral – usually does not cover full expenses.<br>• **Cold weather payments** – £8.50/wk. |

244

**Table 8.3 Benefits for disability and illness**

| | Eligibility | How to apply | Amount |
|---|---|---|---|
| *Statutory Sick Pay* | • Employee age ≥16y. and <65y.<br>• Incapable of work due to sickness or disability<br>• Earning ≥ NI lower earnings limit<br>• Unable to work ≥4d and <28wk. (inc. days when would not normally work)<br>• Those ineligible may be eligible for incapacity benefit or maternity allowance | Notify employer of illness – self-certification first 7d. (SC2 📖 p.225); Med 3 after that time 📖 p.225 | £70.05/wk. Some employers have more generous arrangements. Paid through normal pay mechanisms. |
| *Employment and Support Allowance (ESA)* | • Age ≥16y and < 60y (woman) or <65y (man)<br>• Not entitled to statutory sick pay<br>• Unable to work due to sickness or disability – SC1 certification for first 7d then Med3 certification until work compatibility assessment (done <13 wk into period of sickness/disability) – p. 224<br>• Not receiving income support, income based Job Seeker's Allowance or Pension Credit.<br>**2 types of ESA**<br>• *Contributory ESA* – paid if sufficient NI contributions (unless unfit for work under the age of 20 (25 if in full time education)<br>• *Income related ESA* – full rate is paid if savings ≤£16,000 and income is less than a minimum income; reduced rates may be payable if income is greater than this minimum amount. | Claim from www.jobcentreplus.gov.uk or 0800 055 6688 (textphone: 0800 023 4888) | *First 3d* – no payment<br>*Assessment phase (>3d but <14wk)*<br>• <25y – up to £47.95<br>• >25y – up to £60.50<br>*Main phase (≥14wk)*<br>• Work related activity group – up to £84.50<br>• Support group – up to £89.50<br>🔵 Figures are for a single person. Additional payments may be available for dependents if receiving income-related ESA |
| *Community care grant* | • Receiving Income Support or income-based JSA *and* want to<br>• Re-establish or help the applicant or a family member stay in the community<br>• Ease exceptional pressure on the applicant or a family member<br>• Help with certain travel costs | Form SF300 from local social security offices or ⌨ www.dwp.gov.uk | Minimum payment £30. No maximum amount. |

🔵 Incapacity Benefit – Since 27.10.2008, ESA has replaced Incapacity Benefit for new claims. Those people already receiving Incapacity Benefit will continue to do so at present.

245    CHAPTER 8 **Benefits available**

**Table 8.3** Contd.

| | Eligibility | How to apply | Amount |
|---|---|---|---|
| Disability living allowance (DLA)▽ | • Disability >3mo. and expected to last >6mo. more*<br>• <65y. at time of application<br>**Mobility component:** Help needed to get about outdoors<br>• _Higher rate_ – unable/virtually unable to walk (aged >3y.)<br>• _Lower rate_ – help to find way in unfamiliar places (aged >5y.)<br>**Care component:** Help needed with personal care<br>• _Lower rate_ – attention/supervision needed for a significant proportion of the day or unable to prepare a cooked meal<br>• _Middle rate_ – attention/supervision throughout the day or repeated prolonged attention or watching over at night<br>• _Higher rate_ – 24h. attention/supervision throught day or terminal illness* | ☎ 0800 882200 (0800 220674 in Northern Ireland) or<br>Leaflet DS704 available from Post Offices or<br>Using claim packs available at Citizen's Advice Bureau (CAB) and social security offices or<br>🖥 www.direct.gov.uk | **Mobility component**<br>_Higher rate_ – £46.75/ wk.<br>_Lower rate_ – £17.75/ wk.<br>**Care component**<br>_Higher rate_ – £67.00/wk.<br>_Middle rate_ – £44.85/wk.<br>_Lower rate_ – £17.75/wk. |
| Attendance allowance (AA)▽ | • Disability >3mo. and expected to last >6mo. more*<br>• Aged ≥65y.<br>• Not permanently in hospital or accommodation funded by the local authority<br>• Needs attention/supervision – higher rate if 24-hour care required/terminal illness* | ☎ 0800 882200 (0800 220674 in Northern Ireland) or<br>Leaflet DS704 available from Post Offices or<br>🖥 www.direct.gov.uk | _Lower rate_ £44.85<br>_Higher rate_ £67.00 (for people who need day and night care or are terminally ill) |

▽ No need to receive help to apply. Not means tested.

* Terminal illness (not expected to live >6mo.) – claim under Special Rules. Claims are processed much faster and the highest care rate is automatically awarded. GP or hospital specialist fills in form DS1500 to provide clinical information to support application (fee can be claimed).

| | | | |
|---|---|---|---|
| Disabled facilities grant | For work essential to help a disabled person live an independent life. Means tested. | Apply via local housing department. | Any reasonable application for funds is considered |
| Carer's allowance | • Aged ≥16y; and<br>• Spends ≥35h./wk. caring for a person with a disability who is getting AA or constant attendance allowance or middle or higher-rate care component of DLA; and<br>• Earning ≤ £84.00/wk. after allowable expenses<br>• Not in full-time education | Complete form in leaflet DS700 available from local social security offices or ◼ www.dwp.gov.uk | £46.95/wk.<br>Plus additions for dependants.<br>(➊ No new claims for dependent children have been accepted since April 2003) |

➊
• People who need help to get out of their house are entitled to free prescriptions.
• *Severe disablement allowance is still paid to those who applied prior to April 2001.*

## Table 8.4 Mobility for elderly and disabled people

Local public transport schemes also exist

| | Eligibility | How to apply | Benefits gained |
|---|---|---|---|
| Blue badge scheme | • Age >2y. and ≥1 of the following<br>• War pensioner's mobility supplement<br>• Higher rate of the mobility component of DLA<br>• Motor vehicle supplied by a Government Health department<br>• Registered blind<br>• Severe disability in both upper limbs preventing turning of a steering wheel<br>• Permanent and substantial difficulty walking | Apply through local social services department.<br>● In most circumstances the disabled person does not have to be the driver. The badge should not be used if the disabled person is not in the car.<br>🖳 www.dft.gov.uk | • Entitles holder to park<br>• In specified disabled spaces<br>• Free of charge or time limit at parking meters or other places where waiting is limited<br>• On single yellow lines for up to 3h. (no time limit in Scotland) |
| Motability scheme | • Higher rate mobility component of DLA or<br>• War pension mobility supplement<br>● Driver may be someone else. | Contact motability. Application guide available at<br>🖳 www.motability.co.uk | Registered Charity. Mobility payments can be used to lease or hire-purchase a car, powered scooter, or wheelchair. Grants may also be available for advance payments, adaptations, or driving lessons. |
| Road tax exemption | • Higher rate mobility component of DLA or<br>• War pension mobility supplement or<br>• Person nominated as someone who regularly drives for a disabled person or<br>• Certain types of powered invalid carriages | Usually received automatically. If not and claiming DLA<br>☎ 0845 7123456. If claiming War pension ☎ 0800 1692277 | Exemption from Road Tax |

**Table 8.5 Adaptations and equipment for elderly and disabled people ● All purchases related to disability are VAT exempt**

| | Eligibility | Applying | Benefits received |
|---|---|---|---|
| Occupational therapy (OT) assessment | All elderly or disabled people | Request needs assessment by occupational therapist via local social services department | Enables provision of equipment and adaptations necessary to maintain an independent lifestyle. |
| Disabled Living Centres/Disability Living Foundation | All elderly or disabled people | 49 **Disabled Living Centres** in the UK – list available at ⌨ www.dlcc.co.uk **Disabled Living Foundation:** ⌨ www.dlf.org.uk | **Disabled Living Centres** – Look at and try out equipment with occupational therapists on hand to advise. **Disabled Living Foundation** Information on aids and adaptations |
| Talking books | Anyone with visual impairment | Via the RNIB ☎ 0845 762 6843 ⌨ www.rnib.org.uk – cost of subscription may be paid by local authority. | Talking book library service |
| Telephone | People who have physical difficulty using the telephone or communication problems | British Telecom produce a booklet 'Communication solutions' obtainable from ☎ 0800 800150 or ⌨ www.bt.com If difficulty using a telephone directory register to use directory enquiries free ☎ 0800 5870195 | Gadgets and services that make it easier for disabled or elderly people to use the telephone. |
| Alarm systems | Any disabled or elderly person who is alone at times, at risk, and mentally capable of using an alarm system | Arrange via local social services or housing department. Alternatively, charities for the elderly have schemes (Age Concern – Aid-Call ☎ 0800 772266). | Enables a call for help when the phone cannot be reached. |

● The Royal National Institute for the Blind (RNIB) provides information on low visual aids and other aids and appliances for blind and partially sighted people. They also have an online shop.

# Care of informal carers

In the UK there are 6 million informal carers who are vitally important to the well-being of disabled people in the community. Most are relatives or friends of the person being cared for. Many are elderly with health problems themselves. There is good evidence their health suffers as a result of caring – 52% report treatment for a stress-related illness since becoming a carer and 51% report being physically injured as a result of caring.

GPs and their primary care teams are often the 1st point of access for any help needed and 88% of carers have seen their GP in the past 12mo. Carers see the GP as the professional most able to improve their lives but few GPs have had any training about their problems and 71% carers believe their GPs are unaware of their needs.

**Physical help:** Record whether a patient is a carer in their notes.
- *Practical advice on nursing skills* – ask DNs to review problems.
- *Advice on management* – specialist nurses (e.g. CPNs etc.) provide special expertise.
- *Additional help* – social services can provide home care. Voluntary organisations provide sitting services e.g. Crossroads schemes. Every carer has a right to ask for a full assessment of their needs by the social services.
- *Home modification* – local authorities can arrange modifications. DNs have access to equipment needed for nursing. The Red Cross loans commodes, wheelchairs etc.
- *Respite* – hospitals, charity organisations and local authorities provide day care (to give regular breaks each week) and respite care (for a week or more at a time).

## Emotional support:
- *Self-help carers groups* – opportunity to share experiences with people in similar situations.
- *Always ask the carer how they are when visiting* – even if they are not your patient themselves.
- *If the patient and/or carer have a religion, the clergy will often provide ongoing support*.
- *Maintain good lines of communication*. Treat the carer as a team member. Make sure you inform both carer and patient fully. Make appointments for review. Don't be short with a carer, patronising or impossible to contact.

**Financial support:** Many patients who have carers are entitled to Attendance Allowance or Disability Living Allowance (📖 p.246). If the patient is not expected to live >6mo. they are entitled to claim under Special Rules. This benefit is not means tested. Other benefits:
- *Low income* – 📖 pp.242–4
- *Given up work to look after the patient* – may be eligible for carers allowance – 📖 p.247.
- *Substantial modification to home* – council tax may be payable at lower rate (consult local council).

## Advice for patients: Support organizations for carers

**Carers UK** – ☎ 0808 808 7777 🖥 www.carersuk.org.uk
**Princess Royal Trust for Carers** – ☎ 0844 800 4361
🖥 www.carers.org
**Support organisations for the patient's condition** (e.g. Arthritis Foundation)
**Department of Work and Pensions** 🖥 www.direct.gov.uk/carers
☎ *Benefits Enquiry Line* – 0800 882200; 0800 243355 (minicom facility); 0800 441144 (for help with form completion).
**Citizens Advice Bureau** 🖥 www.adviceguide.org.uk
**Age Concern:** ☎ 0800 00 99 66 🖥 www.ageconcern.org.uk
**Counsel and Care** ☎ 0845 300 7585 🖥 www.counselandcare.org.uk

### GMS contract

| | | |
|---|---|---|
| *Management Indicator 9* | The practice has a protocol for the identification of carers and a mechanism for the referral of carers for social services assessment | 3 points |

### GP tip: Case Skills

A carer skills cause has been developed by Caring with Confidence. Further information is available at 🖥 www.caringwithconfidence.net

## Chapter 9

# The General Medical Services (GMS) contract

# The General Medical Services (GMS) contract

Although there may be some differences in process in each of the four countries of the UK, the principles of the GMS contract apply to all. A total sum for GMS services is given to each primary care trust (PCO) as part of a bigger unified budget allocation. PCOs are responsible for managing the GMS budget locally.

**The Contract:** Made between an individual practice and a PCO. All the partners of the practice, at least one of whom must be a GP, have to sign the contract. It includes:

- National terms applicable to all practices (the 'Practice Contract')
- Which services will be provided by that practice i.e.
  - Essential
  - Additional – if not opted out
  - Out-of-hours (OOH) – if not opted out
  - Enhanced – if opted in
- Level of quality of essential and additional services that the practice 'aspires' to
- Support arrangements e.g. IT, premises
- Total financial resources i.e. global sum + quality achievement payments + enhanced services payments + premises + IT + dispensing

**Essential services:** All practices must undertake these services. *Include:*

- *Day-to-day medical care of the practice population:* health promotion, management of minor and self-limiting illness and referral to secondary care services and other agencies as appropriate.
- *General management of patients who are terminally ill*
- *Chronic disease management*

**Additional services:** Services the practice will usually undertake but may 'opt out' of. If the practice opts out, the PCO takes responsibility for providing the service instead. The practice then receives a ↓ global sum payment.

**Enhanced services:** Commissioned by the PCO and paid for *in addition* to the global sum payment. 3 types:

- *Directed enhanced services:* services under national direction with national specifications and benchmark pricing which all PCOs must commission to cover their relevant population.
- *National enhanced services:* services with national minimum standards and benchmark pricing but not directed (i.e. PCOs do not have to provide these services).
- *Services developed locally:* to meet local needs (local enhanced services) e.g. enhanced care of the homeless.

## Table 9.1 Payment under the GMS Contract

| Payment | Explanation |
|---|---|
| The global sum | Major part of the money paid to practices. Paid monthly and intended to cover practice running costs. <br><br> *Includes provision for:* <br> • Delivery of essential services and additional/ out of hours services if not opted out <br> • Staff costs <br> • Career development <br> • Locum reimbursement (e.g. for appraisal, career development, and protected time) |
| Aspiration payments | Advance payments to allow practices to develop services to achieve higher quality standards. <br><br> Aspiration payments are made monthly alongside global sum payments and amount to roughly 60% of the points achieved the previous year. |
| Achievement payments | Payments made for the practice's achieved number of points in the quality and outcomes framework (📖 p.256) as measured at the start of the following year. <br><br> Aspiration payments already received are deducted from the total i.e. payment for actual points less aspiration pay. |
| Payment for 'extra' services | Paid to practices that provide directed enhanced services, national enhanced services and/or local enhanced services to meet local needs. |
| Minimum practice income guarantee (MPIG) | Protects those practices that lost out under the redistribution effect of the new resource allocation formula. <br><br> Calculated from the difference between the global sum allocation (GSA) under the new GMS Contract and the global sum equivalent (GSE) – the amount the practice would have earned for providing the same service under the old GMS Contract ('The Red Book'). <br><br> If GSA < GSE a correction factor (CF) will be applied as long as necessary so that GSA + CF = GSE. |
| Other payments | Payments for premises, IT and dispensing (dispensing practices only) |

🕐 The Carr–Hill allocation formula is a GMS resource allocation formula for allocating funds for the global sum and quality payments. The formula takes the practice population and then makes a series of adjustments based on the profile of the local community, taking account of determinants of relative practice workload and costs.

# The quality and outcomes framework

The quality and outcomes framework (QOF) was developed for the GMS contract but there are similar arrangements for those working with other contracts. Financial incentives encourage high quality care.

**The domains:** The QOF is divided into 4 domains:
- Clinical
- Organizational
- Additional services
- Patient experience

See Table 2.3

**Indicators:** Every domain has a set of "indicators" relating to quality standards that can be achieved within that domain. The indicators are developed by expert groups based on best available evidence and are updated regularly. All data should available from practice clinical systems. Indicators are split into 3 different types:
- *Structure* e.g. is a disease register in place?
- *Process:* e.g. is a particular measure being recorded? Is action being taken where appropriate?
- *Outcome:* e.g. how well is the condition being controlled?

**Quality points:** All achievement against quality indicators converts to points. Each point has a monetary value.
- *Yes/no indicators:* Points are awarded only if the result is +ve.
- *Range of attainment:* For most clinical indicators it is not possible to attain 100% results, so a range of satisfactory attainment is specified. Minimum standard is usually 40%. Points are allocated in linear fashion by comparison of attainment against the maximum standard e.g. if the maximum is 90%, the minimum 40% and the practice achieves 65%, the practice receives 25/50 (i.e. ½) of the available points.
- *Minimum standard:* All points are awarded if the criterion is met in more than a certain % of cases.

**Exception reporting:** Prevents practices being penalized when unable to meet targets due to factors beyond their control e.g. patients fail to attend for review, or medication is contraindicated. It applies to indicators where level of achievement is determined by % of patients reaching the designated level. Practices report number of exceptions for each indicator set and individual indicator. Ensure the reason why a patient has been 'excepted' from the QOF is identifiable in the clinical record.

**Reporting on quality:** Annually each practice completes a standard return form recording achievement in the past year. Most practices use the Quality and Outcomes Framework Management and Analysis System (QMAS) to do this. There is also an annual quality review visit by the PCO. Based on achievement, the PCO confirms level of achievement funding attained and discusses points the practice will "aspire" to the following year. The process is confirmed in writing and signed off by both parties. PCO-wide quality is checked against other PCOs countrywide.

**QMAS:** Software developed for the GMS Contract in England to allow practices to continually assess their achievement under the Contract and contribute to the calculation of national disease prevalence. Similar software is available for use in Scotland, Wales and Northern Ireland.

## Table 9.2 Calculation of points for quality framework payments

| Components of total points score | Points | Way in which points are calculated |
|---|---|---|
| Clinical indicators | 697 | Achieving pre-set standards in management of: |
| Organizational | 167.5 | Achieving pre-set standards in: <br> • Records and information about patients <br> • Information for patients <br> • Education and training <br> • Medicines management <br> • Practice management |
| Additional services | 44 | Achieving pre-set standards in: <br> • Cervical screening <br> • Child health surveillance <br> • Maternity services <br> • Contraceptive services |
| Patient experience | 91.5 | Achieving pre-set standards in: <br> • Patient survey* <br> • Consultation length |
| **Total possible** | **1000** | |

Clinical indicators — Achieving pre-set standards in management of:
- Asthma
- Atrial fibrillation
- Cancer
- Chronic kidney disease
- COPD
- Dementia
- DM
- Epilepsy
- Heart failure
- Hypertension
- Hypothyroidism
- Learning disability
- Mental health
- Obesity
- Stroke and TIA
- Palliative care
- Primary prevention of CVD
- Smoking

* Improving Patient Questionnaire (IPQ – charge payable) – 🖳 www.cfep.co.uk or General Practice Assessment Questionnaire (GPAQ) – 🖳 www.gpaq.info

In 2007/8 the average value of 1 point = £124.60

## Further information:
**DH** The GMS Contract. 🖳 www.dh.gov.uk
**BMA** The Quality and Outcomes Framework and supporting documents 🖳 www.bma.org.uk
**NHS Employers** 🖳 www.nhsemployers.org
**QMAS** 🖳 www.qmas.nhs.uk

# Exception reporting

Exception reporting allows practices to pursue the quality improvement agenda and not be penalized when they can't meet the quality standards through no fault of the practice, or if meeting the criteria would be inappropriate in the context of a particular patient.

**Reporting:** Practices should report the number of exceptions (Box 9.1) for each indicator set and individual indicator. Exception codes have been added to systems by suppliers. Practices will not be expected to report why individual patients are exceptions but must be able to justify all exceptions with evidence from the patient records if asked to do so.

**Calculation of percentages:** Where there has been exception reporting (Box 9.1), exceptions are subtracted from the number on the register of patients with a particular condition in order to calculate the percentage.

**For example:** A practice has 220 patients on its coronary heart disease (CHD) register of whom 60 have heart failure (HF). 40 patients have been called for routine follow up on 3 occasions in the past year but have not attended. 5 patients have terminal illnesses which make tight treatment targets inappropriate – none of these patients are on the HF register. 2 patients with HF and left ventricular dysfunction can't tolerate ACE inhibitors or angiotensin receptor blockers.

*Sample targets:*
- CHD 1 – register of patients with CHD
- HF 1 – register of patients with HF
- CHD 5 – % of patients with CHD who have a record of BP in the past 15mo.
- CHD 6 – % of patients with CHD who have a record of BP ≤150/90 in the past 15mo.
- HF 3 – % of patients with a diagnosis of CHD and LVD who are currently treated with ACE inhibitors (or angiotensin receptor blockers).

*Reporting:*
CHD 1 – number of patients on the CHD register = 220
HF 1 – number of patients on the LVD register = 60
CHD 5 – 175 patients have a BP record in the past 15mo. but none of those who have not attended follow up.
% of patients who have had a BP record (CHD 5) = $175 \div (220 - 40)$
$$= 97\%$$

CHD 6 – of the 175 with recorded BPs, 160 have BPs within the target range but 2 of those outside the target range have terminal illnesses and a decision has been made and recorded that pursuance of 'ideal' BP is inappropriate.
% of patients who have a BP recorded in the target range
$$= 160 \div (220 - 40 - 2)$$
$$= 90\%$$

HF 3 – 60 patients with HF have LVD – 46 are taking ACE inhibitors – 2 cannot tolerate medication.
% of patients on ACE inhibitors = $46 \div (60-2)$
$$= 79\%$$

## Box 9.1 Valid exceptions

- Patients who refuse to attend review who have been invited ≥3x in the preceding 12mo. (there must be a record of this).
- Patients for whom it would not be appropriate to review the chronic disease due to particular circumstances e.g. terminal illness, extreme frailty.
- Patients newly diagnosed within the practice or who have recently registered with the practice, who should have measurements made in <3mo. and delivery of clinical standards (e.g. BP or cholesterol measurement within target levels) in <9mo.
- Patients on maximum tolerated doses of medication whose levels remain sub-optimal.
- Patients for whom prescribing a medication is not clinically appropriate e.g. due to allergy, another contraindication or adverse reaction.
- Where a patient has not tolerated medication.
- Where a patient does not agree to investigation or treatment (informed dissent), and this has been recorded in their medical records.
- Where the patient has a supervening condition which makes treatment of their condition inappropriate e.g. cholesterol reduction where the patient has liver disease.
- Where an investigative service or secondary care service is unavailable.

# Out-of-hours (OOH) services

Out-of-hours (OOH) is defined as 6.30pm to 8.00am on weekdays, the whole weekend, Bank Holidays and public holidays. Since December 2004, PCOs have taken full responsibility for making sure there is effective OOH provision in the UK.

**'Opting out' of OOH:** Both PMS and GMS practices can 'opt out' of providing an OOH service. The decision must be made for the whole practice – individual doctors within a practice cannot 'opt out' alone. The cost of opting out for a practice is 7% of the global sum (or PMS equivalent).

### Choice of OOH provider:

- PCOs can consider a range of alternative OOH care providers as long as accreditation standards are met. Only where a practice is exceptionally remote can the PCO require a practice to continue providing OOH care. Special arrangements for payment then exist.
- At present, several schemes for OOH cover operate side by side (Box 9.2). For patients housebound with chronic illness or in the terminal phase of disease OOH provision can be unsatisfactory and a lack of communication and continuity of care can result in inappropriate treatment or admissions.

**Communication:** With a variety of agencies involved in provision of OOH cover, good communication between the patient's regular GP and the OOH provider is essential. A universal electronic record for each patient, which can be accessed by any NHS provider, will go a long way towards better communication between providers but until such records are available the onus is on providers to communicate with each other[c].

- If the practice undertakes its own OOH cover, there needs to be a system to ensure OOH contacts are entered in the clinical record.
- If OOH cover is provided by another organization there needs to be a system for transferring information to the practice, transferring that information into the clinical record and identifying any required follow up.

**OOH provision for patients with terminal illness:** When off duty, doctors should ensure there are arrangements which 'include effective hand-over procedures and clear communication between doctors'. It is especially important for patients who are terminally ill or where clinical management is proving difficult.

- If the practice undertakes its own OOH cover, then a system should ensure that all doctors in the practice are aware of these patients.
- If OOH cover is provided by another organization, there should be a system to transfer information from the practice to the OOH provider about patients the attending doctor anticipates may die from a terminal illness in the next few days and may require medical services in the OOH period.

ℹ It is most distressing to bereaved relatives if members of the team do not know of a patient's death. Constructing a procedure to notify relevant members of the primary care team about the death is important.

### Box 9.2 OOH schemes

- **In-practice rotas:** Traditional model of cover. Usually organized in a rota between practice GPs. Largely based on home visiting.
- **Extended rotas:** GPs on-call in rotation for a small group of practices.
- **GP co-operatives:** GPs grouped together (often >100 in a co-op) within a district to cover OOH care between themselves. Often several GPs are on call at any time – one making visits; one taking calls; one seeing patients in a central clinic.
- **Hospital-based OOH cover:** GPs and primary care nurses in A&E departments.
- **Commercial OOH services:** OOH provided by a commercial profit-making organization employing GPs and specialist nurses.
- **NHS Direct:** 24h. nurse-led telephone advice service available throughout the UK. It is designed as a first-line service and aims to have links to local primary care and OOH services. There is also an NHS Direct website and advice booths in public places.
- **NHS walk-in centres:** Walk-in clinics tend to offer nurse consultation and use NHS Direct algorithms. Most are sited in urban areas. They aim to provide easier access to medical care and are increasingly used to cover the OOH period.
- **Enhanced paramedic services:** Providing initial assessment of patients who are not able to get to OOH centres and/or patient transport to OOH centres.
- **Enhanced community nursing teams:** Providing care to patients terminally ill and initial assessment of patients who do not feel able to get to an OOH centre for other reasons.

| GMS Contract | | |
|---|---|---|
| Records 3 | The practice has a system for transferring and acting on information about patients seen by other doctors out of hours | 1 point |
| Records 13 | There is a system to alert the OOH service or duty doctor to patients dying at home | 2 points |

### GP Notes: Improving OOH communication for terminally ill patients

- Leave a written medical summary and medication chart at the patient's home for any health care professional to access should the need arise.
- Provide the OOH provider with a list of patients who may need more intensive support should they call ± directions on management ± a contact number for the OOH provider to call for advice should the need arise.

# Relevant quality indicators

**Palliative care:** 6 points out of a total of 1000 are available for palliative care. In order to achieve these points practices must maintain a register of all patients in need of palliative care or support (palliative care 1) and review all those on the register at a multidisciplinary meeting at least every 3mo.. The definition is broad, so know your inclusion/exclusion criteria and be prepared to justify them.

**Cancer indicators:** Many patients with terminal illness have cancer. The cancer indicators require the practice to keep a record of patients diagnosed with cancer since 1st April 2003, excluding those diagnosed with non-melanotic skin cancer (Cancer 1) and to ensure patients' support needs are reviewed within 6mo. of the practice receiving confirmation of diagnosis (Cancer 3).

**Medication:** Many patients with chronic pain or terminal illness take medication over long periods of time. They are often cared for by a multidisciplinary team with more than one agency initiating and prescribing medication. *It is important that:*

• The notes have a clear indication of when the drug was started and what it was prescribed for (Records 9).
• Any drug allergies/adverse reactions are clearly recorded (Records 8).
• Regular review of repeat medication is carried out (Medicines 11 and 12).

**Carers:** Many patients with chronic pain or terminal illness are looked after by informal carers. As a result of their caring role, many carers develop physical and mental health problems. Identifying and supporting them (Management 9) can help maintain carer health and keep patients in the community for longer.

**OOH cover:** 📖 p.260

**Significant event audit (critical event monitoring):** Recognized methodology for reflecting on important events in a practice. Practices undertaking significant event audit are eligible for quality points (Education indicators 2 and 7). Discussion of specific events can:

• Identify learning objectives *and*
• Provoke emotions that can be harnessed to achieve change.

For it to be effective, it must be practised in a culture that avoids blame and involves all disciplines. Three steps:

• *Decide on a topic and plan a meeting.* A list of suitable events can be made for an individual practice or a pre-formed list of suitable events is available from the Royal College of General Practitioners (RCGP) (Significant Event Auditing: Occasional Paper 70, 1995). Suitable events include new cancer diagnoses and deaths where palliative care has taken place at home.
• At the end of the discussion, *come to a decision* about the case e.g. well managed, need change in procedure etc.

*Prepare a report.* The two acceptable formats for formatting these reports are described in Table 9.4.

## Table 9.3 Relevant QoF indicators

| Indicator | Description | Points | Payment stages |
|---|---|---|---|
| Palliative care 1 | The practice has a complete register of all patients in need of palliative care/support | 3 | |
| Palliative care 2 | The practice has multidisciplinary case review meetings at least every 3mo. where all patients on the palliative care register are discussed | 3 | |
| Cancer 1 | The practice can produce a register of all cancer patients, excluding non-melanotic skin cancer, from 1.4.2003. | 5 | |
| Cancer 3 | % of patients with cancer, diagnosed <18mo. ago who have a patient review recorded as occurring <6mo. after the practice received confirmation of diagnosis | 6 | 40–90% |
| Records 8 | There is a designated place for the recording of drug allergies and adverse reactions in the notes and these are clearly recorded. | 1 | |
| Records 9 | For repeat medicines, an indication for the drug can be identified in the records (if added from 1.4.2004). | 4 | Minimum 80% |
| Medicines 11 | A medication review is recorded in the notes in the preceding 15mo. for all patients being prescribed ≥4 repeat medicines. | 7 | Minimum 80% |
| Medicines 12 | A medication review is recorded in the notes in the preceding 15mo. for all patients being prescribed repeat medicines. | 8 | Minimum 80% |
| Education 7 | The practice has undertaken ≥12 significant event reviews in the past 3y. which could include:<br>• Deaths occuring in the practice premises<br>• New cancer diagnoses<br>• Deaths if terminal care has taken place at home<br>• Suicides<br>• Admissions under the Mental Health Act<br>• Child protection cases<br>• Medication errors<br>• Events in which a patient may have been subjected to harm, had circumstances/outcome been different | 4 points for 12 reviews | |
| Education 10 | The practice has undertaken ≥3 significant event reviews within the last year | 6 points for 3 reviews | |

## Table 9.4 Methods of reporting significant event audits

| Reporting method 1 | Reporting method 2 |
|---|---|
| *Description of event* – Brief. Can be in note form.<br>*Learning outcome* – Aspects of high standard and those which could be improved. Where appropriate include why the event occurred.<br>*Action plan* – The decision(s) taken. Describe reasons for decisions together with any other lessons learned from the discussion. | *What happened?*<br>*Why did it happen?*<br>*Was insight demonstrated?*<br>*Was change implemented?* |

# Additional and enhanced services

**Minor surgery as an additional service:** Includes curettage and cautery and, in relation to warts, verrucae and other skin lesions, cryo-cautery. In all cases, a record of consent of the patient to treatment and a record of the procedure itself should be kept. Payment is included within the global sum payment. If a practice does not want to provide this service it must 'opt out' and the global sum payment is ↓ by 0.6%.

**Minor surgery as a directed enhanced service:** Extends the range of procedures beyond those that practices are expected to do as an additional service. For the purpose of payment, procedures have been divided into three groups:
- Injections – muscles, tendons, and joints
- Invasive procedures – including incisions and excisions
- Injections of varicose veins and piles

**Payment:** Treatments are priced according to the complexity of the procedure, involvement of other staff and use of specialized equipment. Terms for this must be negotiated locally.

**Qualification to provide the service:** Practices can provide this service if they can demonstrate that they have the necessary facilities and personnel (Partner, employee or subcontractor) with the necessary skills. *This includes:*
- Adequate equipment.
- Premises compliant with national guidelines as contained in Health building note 46: General medical practice premises (DoH).
- Nursing support.
- Compliance with national infection control policies – sterile packs from the local surgical supplies department, disposable sterile instruments, approved sterilization procedures etc.
- Ongoing training in minor surgery, related skills, and resuscitation techniques.
- Regular audit and peer review to monitor clinical outcomes, rates of infection, and procedure.

**Minor surgery in PMS practices:** PMS Contracts are negotiated on an individual basis with the local PCO. In most cases, however, the Contract provides for similar arrangements and payments to those in place for GMS practices.

**Influenza and pneumococcal immunizations for at-risk groups as a directed enhanced service:** This directed enhanced service aims to provide influenza and pneumococcal vaccination for the elderly and other 'at-risk' groups – including those with many chronic illnesses and terminal disease. Practices DO NOT have preferred provider status for this service.

### Target group for influenza vaccination:
- Patients aged ≥65y. at the end of the financial year.
- Patients suffering from chronic respiratory disease (including COPD and neuromuscular disease e.g. stroke, MS, Parkinson's disease, MND), chronic heart disease, chronic liver disease, chronic renal disease, immunosuppression due to disease or treatment, or diabetes mellitus.
- Patients living in long-stay residential or nursing homes or other long-stay health or social care facilities.
- Carers of people with chronic disability.

### Target group for pneumococcal vaccination:
- Patients aged ≥65y. at the end of the financial year.
- Patients suffering from chronic respiratory disease (including asthma and patients with neuromuscular disease e.g. cerebral palsy, stroke, MS, MND, Parkinson's disease), CHD, chronic renal disease or nephrotic syndrome, chronic liver disease including cirrhosis, immunosuppression due to disease or treatment (including HIV infection at all stages), asplenia or severe dysfunction of the spleen (including homozygous sickle cell disease and coeliac disease), diabetes mellitus, or individuals with CSF shunts.
- Children aged <5y. who have previously had invasive pneumococcal disease.
- Patients living in long-stay residential or nursing homes or other long-stay health or social care facilities.

### Qualifications to provide the service:
- Practices are expected to use a call–recall system identifying those 'at-risk' through existing registers compiled for use within the quality and outcomes framework.
- Practices not participating in the quality and outcomes framework must compile a register to qualify to provide this enhanced service.

### Targets:
- No target has been set for the proportion of 'at-risk' patients given influenza or pneumococcal vaccination.
- A target of 70% has been set for influenza vaccination of patients ≥65y. – however, a fee per vaccination is payable whether or not this target is reached.
- Additional payments are available through the quality and outcomes framework for vaccinating high proportions of 'at-risk' patients against influenza.

### Anticoagulation monitoring as a national enhanced service
This service aims to provide an anticoagulation monitoring scheme in the community for patients started on therapy in secondary care.

**Practices must:**

- Develop a register of anticoagulated patients – this must include name, date of birth, indication for and length of treatment and target INR.
- Proved a call–recall system.
- Educate newly diagnosed patients and provide ongoing information for established patients including provision of a patient-held booklet.
- Create an individual management plan for each patient on the register.
- Refer promptly to other services and relevant support agencies using local guidelines where they exist.
- Review the patient's health at diagnosis and at least annually thereafter including checks for potential complications.
- Keep records of the service provided including all information relating to significant events e.g. hospital admission death, and ensure these records are included in the GP record.
- Provide ongoing training to staff involved.
- Review the scheme annually including internal and external quality assurance for any computer-aided decision-making equipment or near-patient testing equipment used and audit of care of patients including untoward incidents.

⚠️ It is a condition of participation in the scheme that practitioners will give notification within 72h. of the information becoming available to the practition to the PCO clinical governance lead of all emergency admissions or deaths of any patients covered by this service, where such an admission or death is or may be due to usage of the drug(s) in question or attributable to the relevant underlying medical condition. This notification must occur within 72h. of the information becoming available to the GP.

*Funding available*: Fees vary according to whether the blood is taken in the practice or not, the sample is tested in the practice or not, and the dose is monitored by the practice or not. There are four levels of payment. In addition, a fee per home visit for testing is payable.

**More specialized services for patients with MS as a national enhanced service:** This service aims to address proactively the physical health care needs of patients with MS. National enhanced services are services with national minimum standards and benchmark pricing which are not 'directed' (i.e. PCOs do not have to provide these services).

**Practices must:**

- Produce and maintain a register of patients with MS and their carers.
- Establish a lead contact/co-ordinator.
- Regularly assess their patients with MS including physical symptoms, effect of medication and broader health needs (e.g. associated depression, regular eye tests etc.).
- Provide a personal health plan for each patient on the register.
- Liaise with other agencies e.g. secondary care and social services.
- Provide training and support for involved staff about the nature of MS, making the diagnosis, common complications, symptom control, monitoring and when to refer for specialist care.

- Provide carer support.
- Review the service annually including audit of the register and effectiveness of symptom control techniques, reporting on the existence of appropriate care packages, and feedback from patients on the register and their carers using standardized satisfaction questionnaires.

*Funding available:* Annual fee per patient per year. Paid quarterly in arrears.

# Chapter 10

# Useful information and contacts for GPs and patients

# Useful information and contacts for GPs

## General information

Healthtalkonline patient experience database ▭ www. healthtalkonline.org

NHS evidence: Health information resources ▭ www.library.nhs.uk

### Acupuncture – see Complementary therapy

### AIDS – see HIV/AIDS

### Alternative medicine – see Complementary therapy

### Anorexia/cachexia

Cochrane Berenstein & Ortiz *Megestrol acetate for the treatment of anorexia-cachexia syndrome* (2005).

**European Journal of Palliative Care** Macdonald N *Anorexia-cachexia syndrome* (2005) **12** (2) Supplement p. 8–14

### Anticoagulation

SIGN Antithrombotic therapy (1999) ▭ www.sign.ac.uk
**British Journal of Haematology** Guidelines on oral anticoagulation (3rd edition – 1999) **101**: p. 374–387 ▭ www.bcshguidelines.com

### Ascites

**European Journal of Palliative Care** Campbell C *Controlling malignant ascites* (2001) **8** (5) p.187–191

**Palliative Medicine** Stephenson & Gilbert *The development of clinical guidelines on paracentesis for ascites related to malignancy* (2002) **16** (3) p. 213–8.

### Back pain

**Arthritis Research Campaign** (ARC) ☎ 0870 8505000
▭ www.arc.org.uk

**NICE** Low back pain (2009) ▭ www.nice.org.uk

**New Zealand Screening Questionnaire for psychosocial barriers to recovery** available at ▭ www.nzgg.org.nz

### Cachexia - see anorexia/cachexia

### Chiropractic - see Complementary therapy

### Chronic illness

**BMJ** Von Korff *et al. Organising care for chronic illness.* 2002 (325) 92–94 ▭ www.bmj.com

**The expert patients programme** ▭ www.expertpatients.co.uk

## Chronic obstructive airways disease:

**British Thoracic Society** Spirometry in practice: A practical guide to using spirometry in primary care. 🖳 www.brit-thoracic.org.uk

**RCP/NICE** National clinical guideline on management of chronic obstructive pulmonary disease in adults in primary and secondary care (2004). Thorax 59 (Suppl.1) 1–232.

## Complementary therapy

**Bandolier** 🖳 www.jr2.ox.ac.uk/bandolier/booth/booths/altmed.html

**Effective Health Care.** Acupuncture. 2001 7(2). 🖳 www.york.ac.uk/inst/crd/ehcb.htm

**British Medical Acupuncture Society** ☎ 01925 730727; *Fax:* 01925 730492. 🖳 www.medical-acupuncture.co.uk

**British Acupuncture Council** ☎ 020 8735 0400
🖳 www.acupuncture.org.uk

**Acupuncture Association of Chartered Physiotherapists**
☎ 01747 861151 *Fax:* 01747 861717 🖳 www.aacp.uk.com

**Association of Reflexologists** ☎ 0870 5673320 🖳 www.aor.org.uk

**British Homoeopathic Association** ☎ 0870 444 3950
*Fax:* 0870 444 3960 🖳 www.trusthomeopathy.org

**Society of Homoeopaths** ☎ 01604 621400 *Fax:* 01604 622622
🖳 www.homeopathy-soh.org

**British Homeopathic Library** 🖳 www.hom-inform.org

**Lancet** Linde et al. Are the clinical effects of homeopathy placebo effects? A meta-analysis of placebo-controlled trials (1997) **350** p.834–43.

**British Herbal Medical Association:** ☎ 01202 433691
*Fax:* 01202 417079 🖳 www.bhma.info

**National Institute of Medical Herbalists:** ☎ 01392 426022
*Fax:* 01392 498963 🖳 www.nimh.org.uk

**International Federation of Professional Aromatherapists:**
☎ 01455 637987 🖳 www.ifparoma.org

**Aromatherapy Council:** ☎ 0870 7743477
🖳 www.aromatherapycouncil.co.uk

**Herbmed** 🖳 www.herbmed.org

**British Institute for Allergy and Environmental Therapy**
☎ 01974 241376 🖳 www.allergy.org.uk

**General Osteopathic Council** ☎ 020 7357 6655
🖳 www.osteopathy.org.uk

**British Chiropractic Association** ☎ 0118 950 5950
🖳 www.chiropractic-uk.co.uk

**The Shiatsu Society** ☎ 0845 130 4560 🖳 www.shiatsusociety.org

**The British Wheel of Yoga** ☎ 01529 306 851 🖳 www.bwy.org.uk

**Tai Chi Union** ☎ 0141 810 3482 🖳 www.taichiunion.com

**Chartered Society of Physiotherapy** ☎ 020 7306 6666
🖳 www.csp.org.uk

**UK Pilates Foundation** ☎ 07071 781 859
🖳 www.pilatesfoundation.com

**Pilates Institute** ☎ 020 7253 3177 🖳 www.pilates-institute.com

**Society of Teachers of the Alexander Technique** ☎ 020 7284 3338
🖳 www.stat.org.uk

**British Autogenic Society** ☎ 020 7383 5108
🖳 www.autogenic-therapy.org.uk

**National Federation of Spiritual Healers** ☎ 0845 1232777
🖳 www.nfsh.org.uk

**The Hypnotherapy Association** ☎ 01257 262124
🖳 www.thehypnotherapyassociation.co.uk

**UK Reiki Federation** ☎ 0870 850 2209 🖳 www.reikifed.co.uk

## Constipation
**BMJ** Fallon & O'Neill *ABC of palliative care: Constipation and diarrhoea* (1997) **315** p. 1365–8 🖳 www.bmj.com

## Cough – see breathlessness, cough and stridor

## Counselling
**Psychol Med** Bower *et al* *The clinical effectiveness of counselling in primary care* (2003) 33: 203–15

## Death
### Department of Work and Pensions (DWP)
- **Leaflet D49: What to do after a death in England and Wales**. Available from 🖳 www.dwp.gov.uk/publications/dwp/2006/d49_april06.pdf
- **Funeral payment**: Information and online application form 🖳 www.jobcentreplus.gov.uk

**Scottish Executive** What to do after a death in Scotland. Available from 🖳 www.scotland.gov.uk/Publications/2006/04/12094440/0

## Depression
**DTB** Mild depression in general practice (2003) 4(8) 60–4.

**NICE** Management of depression in primary and secondary care (2004 and update 2007) 🖳 www.nice.org.uk

## Diabetes
**Palliative Medicine** Boyd K *Diabetes mellitus in hospice patients: some guidelines* (1993) **7** p. 163–4

## Diarrhoea
**BMJ** Fallon & Hanks *ABC of palliative care: Constipation and diarrhoea* (2006) **315** 🖳 www.bmj.com

## Disability and benefits

**Department of Work and Pensions (DWP)** 🖳 www.dwp.gov.uk or www.direct.gov.uk/disability

**DWP** Medical Evidence for Statutory Sick Pay, Statutory Maternity Pay and Social Security Incapacity Benefit purposes: A guide for registered Medical Practitioners. IB204 (2004). 🖳 www.dwp.gov.uk/advisers/#med

**Disability Discrimination Act** 🖳 www.disability.gov.uk/disability

**Jobcentre Plus** 🖳 jobcentreplus.gov.uk

## Driving

**DVLA** At a glance guide to the current medical standards of fitness to drive for medical practitioners available from 🖳 www.dvla.gov.uk

Medical advisers from the DVLA can advise on difficult issues – contact: Drivers Medical Unit, DVLA, Swansea SA99 1TU or ☎ 01792 761119

## Drugs

**BNF** 🖳 www.bnf.org

**Medicines and Healthcare products Regulatory Agency** (MHRA – formerly MCA). 🖳 www.mhra.gov.uk

**National Prescribing Centre** A guide to good practice in the management of controlled drugs in primary care (England) (2007) 🖳 www.npc.co.uk

**NHS Business Services Authority** Electronic drug tariff 🖳 www.nhbsa.nhs.uk

**NICE** Medicines adherence (2009) 🖳 www.nice.org.uk

**DTB** Prescribing unlicensed drugs or using drugs for unlicensed applications (1992) **30** p. 97–9

**European Journal of Anaesthesiology** Cohen P *Off-label use of prescription drugs: legal, clinical and policy considerations* (1997) **14** p. 231–50

**Association of Palliative Medicine and Pain Society** The use of drugs beyond licence in palliative care and pain management (2002) 🖳 www.britishpainsociety.org

## Dyspepsia

**NICE** Management of dyspepsia in adults in primary care (2004) 🖳 www.nice.org.uk

## Erectile dysfunction – see sexual health

## Ethics

**Beauchamp & Childress** *Principles of Biomedical Ethics* (5th edition - 2001) OUP ISBN: 0195143329

## Euthanasia

**BBC** Balanced information about the euthanasia debate and links to other sites 🖳 www.bbc.co.uk/religion/ethics/euthanasia

## Flushes – see sweats/flushes

## GP contract

**DoH The GMS Contract.** 🖥 www.dh.gov.uk

**BMA** The Quality and Outcomes Framework and supporting documents 🖥 www.bma.org.uk

**NHS Employers** 🖥 www.nhsemployers.uk

**QMAS** 🖥 www.qmas.nhs.uk

## Headache

**British Association for the Study of Headache** Guidelines for all doctors in the diagnosis and management of migraine and tension type headache (2007) 🖥 www.bash.org.uk

## Heart disease/heart failure

**British Heart Foundation** ☎ 0845 0708 070 🖥 www.bhf.org.uk

**American Heart Association** 🖥 www.americanheart.org

**NICE** Chronic heart failure (2003) 🖥 www.nice.org.uk

Gibbs *et al. ABC of heart failure* (2000) BMJ Publishing. ISBN: 072791457X (❶ new edition due out in 2006)

**NEJM** Digitalis Investigation Group. *The effect of digoxin on mortality and morbidity in patients with heart failure.* (1997) **336**: p.525–9.

**NEJM** Consensus Trial Study Group. *Effects of enalapril on mortality in severe congestive heart failure: results of the North Scandinavian enalapril survival study* (1987) **316**: p.1429–36.

## Herbal medicine – see Complementary therapy

## HIV/AIDS

**British HIV Association** HIV Treatment Guidelines (2003) 🖥 www.bhiva.org

**Health Protection Agency (HPA)** HIV 🖥 www.hpa.org.uk

**Medical Foundation for AIDS and Several Health** HIV in primary care (2004 and revision 2005) 🖥 www.medfash.org.uk

**DoH** Winning ways: reducing healthcare associated infection in England (2004) 🖥 www.dh.gov.uk

## Homeopathy – see Complementary therapy

## Incontinence

**Association for continence advice** Advice for healthcare professionals 🖥 www.aca.uk.com

## Irritable bowel syndrome

**NICE** Irritable bowel syndrome in adults (2008) 🖥 www.nice.org.uk

## Joint and soft tissue injection

**Radcliffe Medical Press** Silver T. *Joint and Soft tissue injection: injecting with confidence* (2001) ISBN: 1857755642

## Lymphoedema

**Cochrane** Badger et al. Physical therapies for reducing and controlling lymphoedema of the limb (2004)

## Motor neurone disease

**NICE** Riluzole for motor neurone disease – full guidance (2001 and review 2004). 🖳 www.nice.org.uk

## Multiple sclerosis

**NICE/RCP** Diagnosis and management of multiple sclerosis in primary and secondary care (2003) 🖳 www.nice.org.uk

**MS Society** A guide to MS for GPs and primary care teams (2006) 🖳 www.mssociety.org.uk

**DoH** HSC 2002/004 Cost effective provision of disease modifying therapies for people with MS 🖳 www.dh.gov.uk

## Nausea and vomiting

**BMJ** Baines M ABC of palliative care: Nausea, vomiting and intestinal obstruction (1997) **315** p. 1148–50 🖳 www.bmj.com

## Organ donation

**NHS Organ Donor Line** ☎ 0845 60 60 400 or sign up on-line at 🖳 www.uktransplant.org.uk

**Blood Transfusion Service** ☎ 0845 7 711 711 🖳 www.blood.co.uk (in South, Mid, East and West Wales ☎ 0800 25 22 66 🖳 www.welshblood.org.uk)

**British Bone Marrow Registry** ☎ 0845 7 711 711 🖳 www.blood.co.uk (in South, Mid, East and West Wales contact the Welsh Bone Marrow Registry ☎ 0800 371 502 🖳 www.welsh-blood.org.uk)

**HM inspector of Anatomy** – whole body donation – ☎ 020 7972 4342/4551

## Osteoarthritis

**Arthritis Research Campaign (arc)** ☎ 0870 8505000 🖳 www.arc.org.uk

**NICE** Osteoarthritis (2008) www.arc.org.uk

## Osteopathy - see Complementary therapy

## Osteoporosis

**NICE** 🖳 www.nice.org.uk
- Osteoporosis – secondary prevention (2005)
- Osteoporosis – primary prevention (2006).

**National Osteoporosis Society** Primary care strategy for osteoporosis and falls (2002) 🖳 www.nos.org.uk

**Royal College of Physicians** Osteoporosis: Clinical guidelines for prevention and treatment (2003) 🖳 www.rcplondon.ac.uk

**RCP (Edinburgh)** Consensus conference on HRT: Final consensus statement (2003) 🖳 www.rcpe.ac.uk/esd/consensus/hrt_03.html

## Pain

**British Pain Society** 🖳 www.britishpainsociety.org
- Recommendations for the appropriate use of opioids in persistant non-cancer pain (2005)
- A practical guide to the provision of chronic pain services for adults in primary care (2004)

**Moore et al.,** Bandolier's Little Book of Pain, OUP 2003, ISBN: 0192632477

**The Oxford Pain Internet Site**
🖳 www.jr2.ox.ac.uk/bandolier/booth/painpag

**World Health Organization** Cancer pain relief: with a guide to opioid availability (1996 – 2nd edition)

**DTB** Opioid analgesics for cancer pain in primary care (2005)

**On-line converter for fentanyl patches**
🖳 www.globalrph.com/fentconv.htm

**Cochrane** – accessed 11/2005 via 🖳 www.nelh.nhs.uk
- Wiffen et al Anticonvulsant drugs for acute and chronic pain
- Saarto & Wiffen Antidepressants for neuropathic pain
- Wiffen et al Carbamazepine for acute and chronic pain
- Wiffen et al Gabapentin for acute and chronic pain
- Li et al Antiviral treatment for preventing post-herpetic neuralgia.

**Bandolier** Topical NSAIDs (2003)
🖳 www.jr2.ox.ac.uk/bandolier/band110/b110–6.html

## Palliative care

**Palliative drugs** 🖳 www.palliativedrugs.com

**Twycross et al** Palliative Care Formulary 2. (2002 – 2nd edition) Radcliffe Medical Press ISBN: 1857755111

**Doyle et al** Oxford Textbook of Palliative Medicine (2005) OUP ISBN: 0198566980

**Dickman et al** The Syringe Driver: Continuous Subcutaneous Infusions in Palliative Care (2nd Edition – 2005) OUP ISBN: 019856693X

**WHO** Definition of palliative care
🖳 www.who.int/cancer/palliative/definition/en

**Woodruff R.** Palliative Medicine. (4th edition – 2004). Oxford University Press ISBN: 019551677X

**NICE** Improving supportive and palliative care for adults with cancer (2004) 🖳 www.nice.org.uk

**Watson et al** Oxford Handbook of Palliative Care, 2nd edition (2009) Oxford University Press ISBN: 0199234356

**Woodruff and Doyle** The IAHPC Manual of Palliative Care (2nd Edition) IAHPC Press (2004) ISBN 0–9758525–1–5
🖳 www.hospicecare.com/manual/IAHPCmanual.htm

**BMJ** Kenyon Z. *Palliative care in general practice* (1995) **311**: p. 888–9
⌨ www.bmj.com

**Gold Standards Framework** ⌨ www.goldstandardsframeworks.nhs.uk

**Princess Alice Certificate in Essential Palliative Care** ☎ 01372 461845
E-mail: education@pah.org.uk
⌨ www.pah.org.uk

**Hospice information** ☎ 0870 903 3903
⌨ www.helpthehospices.org.uk

**SW London and Surrey, West Sussex and Hampshire Cancer Networks** Watson & Lucas *Adult palliative care guidelines* (2006)

## Pelvic pain

**RCOG** ⌨ www.rcog.org.uk
• Management of Acute PID (2003)
• The investigation and management of endometriosis (2000)

## Pressure ulcers

**Tissue Viability Society** Information on bed sores ⌨ www.tvs.org.uk

**NICE** Pressure ulcer management (2005) ⌨ www.nice.org.uk

## Sexual health

**British Heart Foundation Factfile** Drugs for erectile dysfunction (6/2005) available from ⌨ www.bhf.org.uk

**Tomlinson J** *ABC of Sexual Health* (1999) BMJ Publishing ISBN: 0727917595

**Nursing Times** Law C *Sexual health and the respiratory patient* (2001) **97**: NT Plus p. XI–XII

**Oncologist** Penson *et al* *Sexuality and cancer: conversation comfort zone* (2000) **5** p. 336–44

## Steroid cards

• England and Wales: R.R. Donnelley ☎ 0161 683 2390
• Scotland: Banner Business Supplies: ☎ 01506 448 440

## Sweats/flushes

**NEJM** Loprinzi *et al* Megestrol acetate for the prevention of hot flushes (1994) 331(6) p.347–5

**Palliative Medicine** Calder & Bruera *Thalidomide for night sweats in patients with advanced cancer* (2000) **14** (1) p. 77–78.

## Trigeminal neuralgia

**BMJ** Merrison & Fuller *Treatment options for trigeminal neuralgia* (2003) **327** p. 1360–1 ⌨ www.bmj.com

## Vomiting – see Nausea and vomiting

# Information and contacts for patients, relatives, and carers

## General information
**Patient UK** Patient information on a range of topics
🖥 www.patient.co.uk

**Healthtalkonline patient experience database** 🖥 www.healthtalkonline.org

**NHS Evidence Health information resources** 🖥 www.library.nhs.uk

## AIDS – see HIV / AIDS

## Back pain
**The Back Book.** HMSO ISBN: 001 702 0788

**Arthritis Research Campaign** ☎ 0870 8505000 🖥 www.arc.org.uk

## Benefits
**Benefit fraud line** ☎ 0800 85 44 40

**Citizens Advice Bureau** 🖥 www.adviceguide.org.uk

**Department of Work and Pensions** 🖥 www.dwp.gov.uk ☎ *Benefits Enquiry Line* – 0800 882200; 0800 243355 (minicom facility); 0800 441144 (for help with form completion).

**Government information and services** 🖥 www.direct.gov.uk

**HM Revenue and Customs** 🖥 www.hmrc.gov.uk Tax credit enquiry line
☎ 0845 300 3900

**Jobcentre Plus** 🖥 www.jobcentreplus.gov.uk

**Pension service** 🖥 www.thepensionservice.gov.uk

**Veterans Agency** ☎ 0800 169 22 77 🖥 www.veterans-uk.info

## Bereavement
**CRUSE** 0844 477 9400 (young people: 0808 808 1677) 🖥 www.crusebereavementcare.org.uk

**National Association of Widows** ☎ 024 7663 4848
🖥 www.widows.uk.net

## Brain tumour
**Brain and spine foundation** ☎ 0808 808 1000
🖥 www.brainandspine.org.uk

## Cancer
**Macmillan Cancer Support** ☎ 0808 808 2020 🖥 www.macmillan.org.uk

**CancerHelp UK** 🖥 www.cancerhelp.org.uk

## Cardiomyopathy
**Cardiomyopathy Association** ☎ 0800 018 0124
🖥 www.cardiomyopathy.org

## Carers

**Carers UK** ☎ 0808 808 7777 🖵 www.carers.uk.org

**Counsel and Care** ☎ 0845 300 7585 🖵 www.counselandcare.org.uk

**Princess Royal Trust for Carers** ☎ 0844 800 4361 🖵 www.carers.org

**Caring with confidece** 🖵 www.caringwithconfidence.net

**Disability and carers service** 🖵 www.direct.gov.uk/disability or www.direct.gov.uk/carers

## Chronic obstructive pulmonary disease

**British Lung Foundation** ☎ 08458 50 50 50
🖵 www.lunguk.org

## Colostomy

**Colostomy Association** ☎ 0800 328 4257 🖵 www.colostomyassociation.org.uk

## Death

### Department of work and pensions (DWP)

- Leaflet D49: What to do after a death in England and Wales. Available from 🖵 www.dwp.gov.uk/publications/dwp/2006/d49_april06.pdf
- Funeral payment: Information and online application form 🖵 www.jobcentreplus.gov.uk

**Scottish Executive** What to do after a death in Scotland. Available from 🖵 www.scotland.gov.uk/library5/social/waad-00.asp

**Office of Fair Trading**. Arranging funerals. 🖵 www.oft.gov.uk

## Depression

**Depression Alliance** ☎ 0845 123 23 20 🖵 www.depressionalliance.org

## Diabetes

**Diabetes UK**. ☎ 0845 120 2960 🖵 www.diabetes.org.uk

## Disability

**Disabled Living Foundation** ☎ 0845 130 9177 🖵 www.dlf.org.uk

**Citizens Advice Bureau** 🖵 www.adviceguide.org.uk

**Royal Association for Disability and Rehabilitation (RADAR)**
🖵 www.radar.org.uk

**Disablement Information and Advice Line (DIAL UK)** 🖵 www.dialuk.info

**Forum of mobility centres** 🖵 www.mobility-centres.org.uk

**Motability** 🖵 www.motability.co.uk

**Ousiders** 🖵 www.outsiders.org.uk Sex and disability helpline
☎ 0707 499 3527

## Elderly

**Age Concern:** ☎ 0800 00 99 66 🖵 www.ageconcern.org.uk

**Action on Elder Abuse** ☎ 0808 808 8141 🖵 www.elderabuse.org.uk

## Headache

**Organisation for the understanding of cluster headaches (OUCH UK)**
☎ 016 466 51979 🖵 www.ouchuk.org

**Migraine Action Association** ☎ 0116 275 8317 🖵 www.migraine.org.uk

The Migraine Trust ☎ 020 7462 6601 ⌨ www.migrainetrust.org

## Heart disease/heart failure
British Heart Foundation ☎ 0845 0708 070 ⌨ www.bhf.org.uk

American Heart Association ⌨ www.americanheart.org

## HIV/AIDS
NAM Aidsmap ⌨ www.aidsmap.com

National AIDS Helpline ☎ 0800 567 123 (24h. helpline)

Terrence Higgins Trust ☎ 0845 1221 200 ⌨ www.tht.org.uk

## Huntington's chorea
Huntington's disease association ☎ 0151 298 3298
⌨ www.hda.org.uk

## Incontinence
Bladder and Bowel Foundation ☎ 0845 345 0165
⌨ www.bladderandbowelfoundation.org.uk

Spinal Injuries Association ☎ 0800 980 0501 ⌨ www.spinal.co.uk

## Irritable bowel syndrome (IBS)
The Gut Trust ☎ 0872 300 4567 ⌨ www.theguttrust.org

## Lymphoedema
Lymphoedema support network ☎ 020 7351 0090
⌨ www.lymphoedema.org/lsn

UKLymph.com On-line support network ⌨ www.uklymph.com

Skin Care Campaign ⌨ www.skincarecampaign.org

CancerHelp UK ⌨ www.cancerhelp.org.uk

Royal Marsden Hospital ⌨ www.royalmarsden.org.uk

Vascular Society ⌨ www.vascularsociety.org.uk/patient/topics

## Migraine – see headache

## Motor neurone disease
Motor Neurone Disease Association ☎ 08457 626262.
⌨ www.mndassociation.org

Brain and spine foundation ☎ 0808 808 1000
⌨ www.brainandspine.org.uk

## Multiple sclerosis
MS Society ☎ 0808 800 8000 ⌨ www.mssociety.org.uk

Brain and spine foundation ☎ 0808 808 1000
⌨ www.brainandspine.org.uk

### Neuropathic pain
Neuropathy Trust ⌨ www.neurocentre.com

### Organ donation
NHS Organ Donor Line ☎ 0845 60 60 400 or sign up on-line at
⌨ www.uktransplant.org.uk

### Oesophageal cancer
Oesophageal patients' association ☎ 0121 704 9860
⌨ www.opa.org.uk

### Osteoarthritis
Arthritis Research Campaign (arc) ☎ 0870 8505000
⌨ www.arc.org.uk

Arthritis Care ☎ 0808 800 4050 ⌨ www.arthritiscare.org.uk

### Pain
Action on Pain ☎ 0845 603 1593 ⌨ www.action-on-pain.co.uk

Pain concern ☎ 01620 822 572 ⌨ www.painconcern.org.uk

Pain Association of Scotland ☎ 0800 783 6059
⌨ www.painassociation.com

### Parkinson's disease
Parkinson's Disease Society ☎ 0808 800 0303
⌨ www.parkinsons.org.uk

### Pelvic pain
⌨ www.hysterectomy-association.org.uk

⌨ www.womenshealthlondon.org.uk

Pelvic Pain Support Network. ☎ 0845 125 5254 ⌨ www.pelvicpain.org.uk

National endometriosis society ☎ 020 7222 2776.
⌨ www.endo.org.uk

### Sexual problems
Information sheets for patients with disability (SPOD)
☎ 0707 499 3527 ⌨ www.outsiders.org.uk

### Suicide and self-harm
Samaritans 24 h. emotional support via telephone ☎ 08457 90 90 90
⌨ www.samaritans.org

Self injury and related issues (SIARI) ⌨ www.siari.co.uk

Survivors of bereavement by suicide ☎ 0844 561 6855
⌨ www.uk-sobs.org.uk

### Thrombosis
Lifeblood: The thrombosis charity ☎ 0207 663 9937
⌨ www.thrombosis-charity.org.uk

### Trigeminal neuralgia – see also neuropathic pain
Trigeminal neuralgia association UK ☎ 01883 370 214
⌨ www.tna.org.uk

# Index